Praise for
THE WAY WE SLEEP

"*The Way We Sleep* represents the very best of what a book can do that no other narrative medium can touch; it's part anthology, part art-book, part interview, part graphic novel, part confessional, part essay, part sociological study. The subject matter here ranges from sex to family to coming-of-age, all rendered with a delightful wit, brevity, and charm. From Mary Roach's study of insomnia to Tony Millionaire's depiction of epic torpor to the Residents' exploration of sleepwalking, *The Way We Sleep* is as intimate, poignant, and humorous as anything whispered beneath the sheets."

— Joe Meno, author of *Office Girl, The Great Perhaps*
and the best-selling novel *Hairstyles of the Damned*

"At once a hybrid text and a compendium of tales related more or less loosely to the theme of sleep, this generously sized volume edited by C. James Bye and Jessica Bye offers flash-length tidbits and short stories by well-known and less well-known writers, interviews with movie and TV directors, and a healthy dose of comics."

—*Los Angeles Review*

"Here is a wonderful book filled with stories about the one last taboo left in the American bedroom: sleep. Aside from honest and intimate storytelling about the one last fun legal thing left on our landscape, I should advise you that on page 137 of my copy there is an illustration of the grim reaper chasing a young man with a knife. If that last sentence doesn't pique your interest, you're dead or medicated and not interested in what I'm saying here. That's fine; this was either the wake-up call you needed, or the worst book blurb ever. Also, chances are, I'm writing this from your bed. Try not to wake me when you get home."

—Dan Kennedy, host of The Moth storytelling podcast,
author of *Loser Goes First* and *Rock On: An Office Power Ballad*

"Combining mattress-popping humor with writing as fresh as newly-laundered cotton sheets, *The Way We Sleep* will keep you wide awake with reading pleasure." —Dinty W. Moore, author of *The Mindful Writer*

"Let's say you snooze for eight hours every night. I know: dream on. There's finally a book dedicated to the roughly four months you spend under the covers every year. *The Way We Sleep* will keep you up way too late reading just one more charming story or essay or interview or comic strip. Not since Proust has our somnolence been described in such depth." —Andrew Ervin, author of *Extraordinary Renditions*

D1453714

"I can't think of a subject more overdue for a book-length examination than sleep. Co-editors, Jessa and Casey Bye—along with the fine and funny writers and artists they bagged for this collection—poke and prod the bed from every possible angle: the hysterics caused by a sleepless night, the lust and joy and weirdness induced by dreams, and the ridiculous lengths we go to get a good night's rest, all while drawing surprisingly fitting connections to subways, socks, snow storms and superheroes. Reading *The Way We Sleep* is nothing short of a delight, a reminder that few of life's challenges make us more human than the common desire to close our eyes and disappear for a while."

—Richard Nash, founder of Cursor, *Red Lemonade*, former publisher of Soft Skull

"Some beds are small; you have to curl up in them to feel right. Other beds are long and your toes thrill to the absence of limits. Some beds are plush and hard to get out of. Others are rickety and move when you move. These qualities might not always seem ideal for beds, but they're perfect for short stories, comics, and short interviews, as this anthology proves."

—Ben Greenman, author of *The Slippage*

"Fun!"

—Adam Levin, author of *The Instructions*

THE
WAY
WE
SLEEP

THE WAY WE SLEEP

Edited by
C. James Bye and Jessa Bye

Curbside
Splendor

CURBSIDE SPLENDOR PUBLISHING

Published by Curbside Splendor Publishing, Inc., Chicago, Illinois in 2012.

Some of these works previously appeared in the following places:

"The Bed Frame" first appeared in *TriQuarterly*
"Cramps" from *The Girl on the Fridge* by Etgar Keret. Translation copyright © by Etgar Keret. Reprinted by permission of Farrar, Straus and Giroux, LLC.
"Derrick Mickelson's Cuddle Bed for Wayward Boys" first appeared in *Harpur Palate*
"Erika's Dreams" first appeared in the *Seattle Stranger*
"Goodnight Nobody" previously appeared in *Pequin* and *Witness*
"Hands to Work" first appeared in *Corium Magazine*
"Jugs" first appeared in *[PANK] 1*
"Physiological Draught" first appeared in *Prick of the Spindle*
"Sleepless in Suburbia" first appeared in *Reader's Digest*
"Soak" first appeared in *Owen Wilson Review*
"Your Dreams and What They Mean" first appeared in *Monkeybicycle7*

First Edition

Copyright © 2012 by Casey Bye and Jessa Bye

Library of Congress Control Number: 2012951909
ISBN: 978-0-9884804-0-7

Edited by C. James Bye and Jessa Bye
Designed by Steven Seighman
Cover illustrations by Drew Shannon

Manufactured in the United States of America.

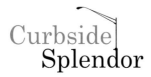

www.curbsidesplendor.com

CONTENTS

EDITORS' NOTE

Our relationship had its genesis in a bed. It's not a salacious story—Jessa had a dream that was vaguely erotic about Casey (if you think that the idea of him begging her to wait until "we are in love!" to have sex is erotic). That led to a Facebook post and slightly more open flirting until we first kissed at a party that Jessa's then-boyfriend was bartending at.

Two Decembers later, we were cohabiting in a lovely Rogers Park apartment and lying in bed, discussing a book idea that Jessa had abandoned a year or so previously. At the time, Casey had recently finished his thesis and Jessa was working at a debt collection law-firm, assisting in lawsuits against people who defaulted on their student loans. We were both long overdue for a new project.

In the following few hours of discussion, this book started to form itself. It wouldn't be a collection of Jessa's short stories any longer (thank goodness for you!)—instead it would be an anthology of varied and talented voices. Instead of being a regular paperback with ten or so stories it would be of honking art book size and accentuated with comics and interviews.

Over the course of planning this book, we've also planned a wedding and moved from Chicago to Memphis. Our lives have changed drastically, but all of those changes were prefaced and shaped by long conversations in bed.

One of the most interesting things we've found during this process is just how aligned we were in our selections. Despite the fact that Casey's magazine (*Knee-Jerk Magazine*) and Jessa's (*Monkeybicycle*) are very

different, we ended up gravitating to the same material. The anthology is about beds and sleep, and as a result you will find this book chock full of magic realism, vulgarity, humor, sentiment, earnestness, conversation, beauty, absurdity, heartbreak and an itty bitty bit of sex. Kind of like your own bed.

Although hopefully not too much heartbreak, because that'd be a downer.

Enjoy!

<3 Jessa & Casey

THE
WAY
WE
SLEEP

PHYSIOLOGICAL DROUGHT

MATTHEW SALESSES

I can hear his hands slapping over his flat stomach from the bathroom, where he is pouring out the buckets of water we've saved for these makeshift showers. At the beginning of the drought, before the city reservoir ran dry, we had filled them up together.

It has been thirty days now of emergency drought, and the three stores in our area have run out of bottled water, so that we have to take the bus to get something to drink. He is singing *Ave Maria* but doesn't know the words and isn't religious. He is getting ready to go look at the house down the street, anticipating the real estate agent I know he has a crush on. How can he not be hungover?

Pushing through the clutter from close to six years together I drag my hangover down the hall to the kitchen. Beer glasses stolen from French cafés, bone china from England, blue condom wrappers, a bucket of paint, art prints from our year in New York. Under the sink are stacks of our books. His *Zen and the Art of Motorcycle Maintenance*, my *Middlemarch*. Dave is Holden Caulfield, Diane is Nicole Diver. When we met I was almost thirty and he was just out of college. The first time he said he loved me I didn't say a word.

The bottles of water he said he would bring home from the restaurant where he cooks are nonexistent. I try to dry-swallow two aspirin but choke them up as they turn to clouds of chalk.

Last night he pulled his meanness out as if

from a pocket and gave it to me, blurred and bleeding, carried a long way, like a note that had gone through the wash.

According to the weatherman New England hasn't had a drought of this severity since the eighteenth century. The clouds refuse to give up their rain, even though they hug each other for room in the crowded sky.

The first week the drought received emergency status we went up to the roof of our apartment building with water balloons, but were too ashamed to throw them at anyone but each other. We stared down to the street we have lived on for four years.

The second week of the drought he told me about the four kinds of drought: meteorological, agricultural, physiological, and hydrological, and said we were in the first, second, and fourth, and the fourth was why the city had shut off our water. I asked what was the third, and he told me the third was when plants for some reason stopped being able to drink.

★ ★ ★

I undress and wait for him to come out of the bathroom and leave me, or for me to leave him. We will walk down the street to this other house, at least. I remember how happy we were when we made this appointment, the second week of the drought. Now we will keep it as if nothing is different, as if the problem were just dehydration from fucking too hard. I will tell him I'm going to talk and he is going to listen and shut up and not fight back. I will tell him a good deal and make him listen until one of us cries.

In just the space between two houses I could end us. All I would have to say is this (I've been saving it up for a year): I told you I needed that baby after all—that seven-pound, two-ounce boy that was suddenly not my body—and it's still true.

I am sorry I told him last night for the first time, which should have been the second. I don't know why I said: You ruined my life and not just mine. What I should have said was: Sometimes things that don't happen change your life as much as things that do.

As we walk I hope he remembers what he said last night, that falling down is just the step before getting back up. What a bastard he is.

I could tell him I wish we had named our child before we let him go. I would have named him Justin. I could have been convinced otherwise. He's over two years old now, far away from this drought. Maybe he wouldn't have survived it had he been here, with us. Maybe we would have saved him our last drops of water, keeping him alive.

If I were braver, I would say: (a) I doubt you'll get over me. And (b) I remember I said I would never marry you; you never brought it up again.

★ ★ ★

We get to the apartment and the real estate agent holds the door for me and Dave holds the door for her. Her name is Joan. She is incorrectly beautiful: all her features are wrong in a way I could point out, but I couldn't deny a sort of attractiveness that any woman would hate. He doesn't let it show that we've been fighting.

He is already on his way to the bedroom, brushing past the space in the entranceway where in our house he would have knocked over the little figurine he got me for our first Valentine's six years ago. I would have spent the next hour cleaning up the shards of Buddha's stomach and thinking of a place to put them where he would roll onto their sharp points. Instead I follow him and the smell of fresh cologne.

From the bedroom window I can see into our little house down the street, the apartment we just left. He digs his toes into the plush because he saw it in *Die Hard*.

Joan is saying, "I think a couple could be very happy here."

I stare out the window to where, in our kitchen, on another day, I might be baking or rummaging around in the knives. I want to tell Joan that we're only here because good people don't break appointments, we're only here because my boyfriend likes her.

"Who lived here before?" I ask.

"A woman with a family."

"Does it matter who lived here before?" he says.

"My head hurts," I say, "I need a glass of water."

He puts his hand on my head. "What's this?" he says.

It's an old joke. "Brainsucker," he will say, "what's it doing? Starving."

I walk out to the kitchen, and Joan yells that the faucet doesn't work, because of the drought, but I try it anyways. A little brown sludge leaks out with what used to be water.

"I told you," she says, without looking.

I look around: three bedrooms, two bathrooms, and a covered-up past. I can see how someone had loved this apartment and then cleaned it and cleared it out to sell. I can see how it still breathes with the stench of their breath.

When I return he's lying on the bed. "It must take a while before someone new buys the place," he's saying. "What happens in the meantime? Is it rented out?"

Joan says the woman who owns it comes back from time to time.

The only dressings to the room now are the maroon drapes, a stained bureau, and the queen-sized bed in the middle where Dave lies, full of his youth in a new house.

I could make this place so cute. I mentally decorate it with all the things that we own, that I own. I don't ask how much, because I know it's out of our price range.

Joan says the furniture that is left stays with the house. "Isn't that bed comfortable?" she says. Dave bounces on it to show her it is.

I say I'm going to walk around to the other rooms. Joan gets ready for me to leave, and I hear them begin to speak as I go.

I find two ice cubes in the freezer that must be from before the drought, and slip them cold into the well of my mouth.

The second week of the drought I started coming home from the flower shop early, before he left for work. He cooked for me four nights in a row, which I knew he hated to do before working. We made an agreement to move to a bigger apartment. He told me stories I had never heard before, like how he traded his coat for the chance to talk with me, the first time we met, to the friend who introduced us.

The third week of the drought fires broke out in the Appalachians and Dave said the water that was left would go to fighting them. He said the worst drought in history had killed five million people in China.

I suck on the ice cubes thinking how the drought has made him more talkative.

Eight hours ago he said he was saying goodbye. I said, "Don't worry, I look my best in rear-view mirrors." One last, clever line. You know, objects in mirror...or am I getting that backwards?

★ ★ ★

Now I think of a morning he wasn't there, when I pushed through the forest of wedding dresses, talking about him and choosing a gown for my sister. Mom was plotting me a chart of his pluses and minuses; Lou was in the dressing room trying on the gowns we chose, snow-covered pines like the big-butted trees Dave and I had seen in the Alps. They had long trains as if winter had forgotten where the tree ended and ground began. I was hunting out the newer dresses and Mom was focused on the old-fashioned ones, which, she said, had come back in style. We had been let in before the store opened as a favor to her current boyfriend who knew the owner.

I was explaining to her about Europe once again, how the mountains were higher and seemed older and about how Vermont meant nothing to me now. I was explaining to her how Dave and I were in it for the long haul.

"You two are really happy," she said.

I told her to stop equivocating. She didn't ask what it meant.

"You know I support you," she said, "but what can he give you?"

Everything to break a heart.

(Later that day, when I said the dresses were all for skinny people, he would hint at how I'd gained weight.)

What could he give me? "You mean other than love?" I said.

We kept shaking the branches of those dresses loose from the rack and handing them into the dressing room. It was early because Mom had to be in to work by nine, and only Lou had any

energy. I felt weak at the belt, and Mom couldn't stop wanting a cigarette, but Lou was an engine sputtering our spare parts into motion. "What about you?" she would say, "When's it your turn?"

"Honey, you got to start thinking about your future," Mom said. "I know you don't think you're old, but your little sister is getting married."

I was aware of that. "I'm thinking about my future," I told her.

"What about this kid says 'wedding?'"

"What about Lou and Jared says wedding? And don't call him a kid."

"I'm just saying the things moms say, you know?" Then she said, "You're starting to show," and I panicked.

Any day I will have to tell her she was right about him, now that she's gotten used to the idea of us together. After everything I said to convince her so I could convince myself. I wonder if he'll want to stay friends, to make it easier on her.

★ ★ ★

The third week of the drought was when I noticed how dry my mouth was getting. Dave said he had a solution, and I sucked him off the way he liked. He bought me hand moisturizers and wrapped them up like presents. He talked about going on vacation. He said they wouldn't let us take liquids on the plane, so a vacation would be perfect for when we were all dried out.

I remember how I brought him to see Mom after the first year passed and we were still all over each other. She took us up to the lake in Maine that my family went to every summer, and he lay in the hammock reading short stories by New Yorkers, laughing once in a while like a whine.

In the evenings we went swimming together: he would kick out from our little dock too hard and pull me along past the places I had wanted to stop and show him. Just things I thought he'd like, like the loon's nest and the mud where in the old days I almost always saw moose tracks.

The third week of the drought he filled the tub with precious water he had saved and heated and we took a bath. The fourth week he said he regretted it.

The fourth week he started to speak in abstractions, saying the drought would go on forever. He made bad jokes, like saying, "I drought it" instead of "I doubt it."

I remember we had fireworks on the lake that summer and he put on a big show and then acted like it was nothing. I could tell Mom was impressed then. I could tell she was thinking he could light up the world for me. I had to make her see how it was worth it to put one baby down as a bet against returns. She wrote me her compliments in list form later that month, right up next to her complaints, bulleted and organized the way she wrote everything she knew she was seeing objectively and I wasn't.

* * *

Now he's in the other room, laughing with another woman. I lie down in this bed next door, head drowning for water. Sinking here I can't help but worry, how will everything be divided if he leaves me? The only way I can think is to smash it all down the middle and leave it in halves. Who's to say the woman Solomon didn't give the baby to would have loved it less? Maybe there were extenuating circumstances, a man, life. Maybe she loved what she had so much she couldn't let anything remain. Halves can be better than all or nothing.

The fourth week of the drought Dave said a person could only live three days without water and one without fun. He painted my nails silver and then made me dance so close I speckled his shirt. The fourth week of the drought he made me fight him, he said he expected me to fight back better than I did.

(I have questions for our future selves. I would ask my future self, do you think of him fondly, so I would know how much I had to ruin those memories now and how much of them I could leave intact. I would ask his, do our stories match, so if they didn't I could set him straight before he leaves.)

I want to ask, do you remember when we went to Europe and I walked around blacked out, for example, missing the fact that we were standing by the Arc de Triomphe, as you told

me afterwards? In the moment you were the attraction I couldn't wait to see. The Dave you talked about being overseas.

If I have to remember I want to remember him like this, the good Dave.

The fourth week of the drought I closed the flower shop—we had no more flowers—and Suzy came over from next door to say hello. She's five years old, twice the age of our baby. Her nanny brought her over. When Suzy hugged me I could feel the parts of him that had grown on me. I offered Suzy a plastic rose, one that would last. Her nanny asked if there wasn't anything real. I shrugged and held the child in my arms.

* * *

But I keep coming back to that day with my mother, my sister getting ready for marriage in the changing room, three years ago. I watched Mom choose an awful dress humped up around the waist, like the one in the picture of her wedding to Dad, and ask please could she see one of her daughters in this. I hadn't eaten yet that morning and felt dizzy.

Mom always said she should burn that picture, but I knew she would keep it, not because she loved the dress, but because a wedding was a wedding. She held a cigarette in her mouth and her lipstick rubbed off on the filter. She couldn't smoke in the shop; she said it was for the oral fixation.

When Lou was ready for a change she would thump on the door and we handed over another gown. We had already gone through what could have clothed a country of brides. I imagined her in there: puffing herself up like a cat seeing its reflection. Back then I could laugh about how we resembled ourselves.

(Sometimes Dave woke me in the night to tell me he'd dreamed I left him for another man. How I was such a bad person in his sleep. He would go back to bed and I would stay up, trying not to listen to his puffing snores. In the morning he would act like I was a whore, and—somehow—I would feel like one.)

I wanted my mother to say I had someone I shouldn't let go of. I gave away the secrets I could: being carried around the little villages in the Alps on Dave's back, long meals of long conversations and lots of the sound of his French, how he took candids of me and how in each one I was smiling as he caught me by surprise.

"He's really that good?" she asked.

"He's really that good."

When I went home Dave was still in bed, sleeping, sitting up like a freak, guarding a dirty house.

Lou shouted that we had forgotten her. We could hear her shift things around, turning the changing room into her closet. "When will there be time?" she asked. "Ma, you got to work in less than an hour. Dave's great. Jared liked him."

Mom whispered to me but I didn't hear. She shoved a couple gowns over the door. She swept through the designers to get to our price range, in the back, like dusting the snow off of interrupting pines.

I wish I had known then how the first week of the drought Dave held me up by my ankles while I drank a glass of water to cure hiccups. The second week he slipped ice cubes down my skin. The third week he took me to the aquarium and dared me to swim with the seals. The fourth week he made a single cup of coffee and left it, empty, by the sink.

Mom started an avalanche of gowns. She was clumsy in the most normal situations, something that surprised people about her.

"You have to listen to me," I said. I thought if I could convince her then we would be real enough to sacrifice for. I wanted to be as permanent as she could make us. By then I would have told her anything to make her love him; she always thought of all my boyfriends as Dad.

"I'm listening."

"You have to listen to me," I said again. We were stumbling over white fabric.

"I'm listening," Mom said. I pictured Dave running off and leaving Mom high and dry.

I thought of Lou not eating for three weeks to fit into these dresses, her fiancé by her side to pick out the china and floral arrangements, things mattering only in the small sphere of a couple tented out in the midst of endless

pine gowns. I looked at photos of prospective families for months and Dave never joined in the adoption.

(The fifth week of the drought he was licking my nipples when Mom called and kept licking while I was talking on the phone. The fifth week of the drought I was home all day and so was he, and I saw for the first time in years how he spent his time doing none of the things I asked. The fifth week of the drought he would wait until it was just before he left for work and then he would try to fuck me.)

"You have to listen," I said. When I gave birth, Mom waited by my bedside holding Dave's hand, and with every scream I wished my pain would bring them closer together, with every scream I knew my baby and I were growing farther apart.

Mom grabbed at the dresses. I reached for a falling white sequined number that had caught my eye like an exploding galaxy, and the sequins fell off in my hands. The beads fell to the floor, some of them settling silently in the folds of the fallen dresses, but most of them scattering with the patter of hail. Lou screamed from the dressing room. I thought we must have been ignoring her thumps again. It wasn't my fault. The dress tore itself up on its own.

"You ruin everything," my sister shouted. "Everything has to be about you. When will there be time? I'm trying to have a wedding."

The fifth week of the drought I realized the fact that we had a baby out there, somewhere in the world, and that my mother knew about it, was why I had stayed with Dave for so long. (Last night he half-fucked me on the bed before taking me out. He held my arms against my back and I let him. Last night he fought with me and was too drunk to make it to bed, and he held me tight to him, and I held him back, on the floor.)

I threw up the entire trip home. Mom took a half-day at work to drive me over the state line back to Massachusetts. On the way I convinced her the adoption was a good idea; I'm not sure how; she didn't want to break my heart. I let myself believe her blessing was all we needed. She drove slowly and let me talk. We pulled over for me to puke over the barrier. She rubbed my stomach as she drove. I felt young; she made me feel young. I stuck my arm out against the seatbelt, keeping it loose. We worried about what to do with the dress; only Mom's boyfriend knew the owner. Nobody had seen. It was a cheap dress and I offered to pay for it or find someone I knew who might want it. I never told Dave about it, and I remember when he yelled about the bill.

★ ★ ★

I love you I

love you I love you.

In my dream, as I put my head down in this other room, and my lips peel back like a flower dying of thirst, we have lived in this house— three bedrooms, two bathrooms—for twenty years. Here on the dresser is the little snow globe of Napoleon. Here over the desk is the map of the world. He sleeps in the bed and I check in on him while frying mushrooms, his favorite, so the aroma will wake him. Here is the chair my father used to rock in; I saved it from Mom's wrath. Here is his mother's portrait that was left him in her will. I will walk from room to room; it takes a lifetime, and in between are the signs that it was good. In the steam on the mirror I will catch a message he left me. Here in the third room is an old crib. There on the couch is the faintest red, from spilled wine, from a fight. First the front hall crumbles into bitten fingernails, then the back wall falls into broken dreams, then the floor opens and everything folds together like his shut eyes. In his dreams tonight I will whisper these sweetest words. From wherever he is then he will hear me in his sleep and know it's me. He will know it's the woman of his best six years. He will hear my words go by, in clusters of three that could have been his: I will pull their strands from my threaded heart so that the next time I say them, forgetting him, I will know that nothing I give is second-hand.

THE EXCELLENT ACTOR DAVID STRATHAIRN

SHARON GOLDNER

Alan and Marlene are making love. In some circles you could say:

They are doing it.

They are screwing their brains out.

They're getting it on.
They're inserting Point A into Point B.
They're making whoopee.

The excellent actor David Strathairn is walking around their bed. He rubs his chin. This kind of action never really gives anyone any answers, and in some circles it could be misperceived as a gesture common to very poor acting. Mr. Strathairn is anything but a poor actor. You may not be able to put a face to his name, but you have seen him in lots of movies and on television, and when you see him you go, "Hey, I know that guy." You just don't know his name. You might know other actors. You know Al Pachino and Robert DeNiro. You might know David Arquette. They're all actors too. They all write it down as occupation on their tax forms. It's a shame if you know David Arquette and not David Strathairn though. Arquette is married to Courtney Cox and she is an actress and she seems sensible enough with her roles and maybe in her marriage too, but the face that you know David Arquette and not David Strathairn is a little creepy. I'm sorry, but David Strathairn is a much better actor. Marlene only recently learned his name. There's no accounting for the order of things some days.

Taking into account the lackluster two on the bed, David Strathairn finally says weakly, "Whoopee." He has made this call and is sticking with it. He doesn't need a script. He doesn't need a director. He is calling it like he is seeing it, and he is that good. David Arquette never could have taken this part.

Marlene sees David Strathairn, not out of the corner of her eye, but out of the whole of her eye. And then the other eye too. She blinks back and forth a couple of times. "Jesus Christ," Marlene says.

Alan, taking the lord's name as a great anticipatory lovemaking sign, gets even more excited.

"No, no. No Jesus Christ, not like that," Marlene says. She hasn't had a Jesus Christ moment with their lovemaking in quite some time. When Alan gets back to the task at hand, Marlene says, "I know you. You're David Strathairn, the excellent actor. I just saw you in a movie."

David Strathairn blushes. It's always nice to be recognized, and this one knows his name. While that may not be a first, it may very well be a third or a fourth. "This, apparently, is my latest role," he says. His voice is like cold sweat, molten and arctic, that ribbons on the fringe of the skin, barely above where one's outline of existence starts and meets with the nothing that comes after us, though air would beg to differ about being called nothing. "I am playing the part of your inner voice."

"So you've always been on the inside?" Marlene asks, curious and just a little unnerved.

"No, not all that long. My agent said, while not the role of a lifetime, it was good for the acting chops, a cut away from the lamb and the veal. I just improvised that you know," so says David S.

"You're very good," Marlene says, Alan huffing and puffing away in the background. "More people should know your name."

"I'm a working actor," David S. says. "It's all okay. Anyway, it was time to come out today and see what's up." He walks around to face Alan, ferocious, no, tired, no, ferociously tired, going at it. "Mentally I think I am prepared. Now, I'm ready to do the legwork—the blocking, the dialogue, the interactions with the others. We're going to get this production underway."

"Wow," Marlene says. "Being a pre-school teacher, nothing exciting really happens to me. I'm lucky if I get through a day when no three year old has made in his pants. Now that's a good day! That is—just—I don't know. Oh my God?"

Alan stops mid-thrust. "No, no, not that oh my God. I'm not finished yet, Alan. One, two, three and he's done," Marlene complains.

"Is he always this inconsequential?" David S. asks. He is on bent knee, examining things from a different angle. "Alan and Marlene: doing the nasty."

Marlene says, "I wish. This is so boring. I mean, it must be boring to you. You're a famous actor. You've won awards."

"Alan and Marlene: getting a piece," says Daivd S., bending his knees to look from the opposite of things.

"Yeah well," Marlene says, "the only piece I'm getting is a piece of charley-horse...down there."

"Alan and Marlene: booty calling and booty doing. Booty charley-horse," David S. says. "Giddy-up."

Marlene asks David Strathairn if he knows everything about her, because being an excellent actor, he clearly immerses himself in his roles which means he has immersed himself in her. "Because if you've done your research," she says, "you would know about the time Alan outfitted me in these really height-worthy spiked heels. They were like if Frankenstein was a drag queen prostitute whore. But who am I to judge someone else's fetish? So I'm wearing them, right, and Alan's on top and I inadvertently lift my leg. I hit him in the scrotum."

David S. Says, "That would be an ouch." Then without missing a beat, he re-writes his own line to "ouch" in a very high voice.

Marlene asks if David S. knows how many ice packs it takes to get a swollen scrotum down. The excellent actor asks if there is a punchline somewhere there, like how many Polocks does it take to get the swelling down on a scrotum?

"No Polocks were involved," Marlene says. "Just Alan and his swollen balls."

David S. points out that Alan's balls are better now, because Alan and Marlene are perpetrating. They're down in the hood. They're all up in each other's business. They're banging each other. Marlene asks the excellent actor to stop; turns out, she's the one with balls. But the actor's got one more.

"No," Marlene says.

David S. promises that it is just one more. "No." He says it is a short-stack one. "No."

"Alan and Marlene are—badunkadunking."

"Okay, you know," Marlene says, "that was so not short. You said short. That was easily five syllables."

"So sue me," David S. says. "I am an excellent actor, not an English major. You are deviating here. We have to get back on task. This doesn't look too good. He clearly doesn't know what he's doing. His hands are all wrong; elbow bending reduces stress. The expression on his face; is that a grimace or is that ecstasy? He's got his right foot in, he's got his left foot out, he's shaking all about. Is he doing the hokey pokey or making love?"

"Okay look," Marlene begins. "At first I thought that maybe this was going to be cool. There's an actor in the bedroom and he's famous and successful and he is in his current role as *my* inner voice. I wasn't even aware there were auditions. But now that we're at this place, I must say this feels wrong on so many levels."

The most excellent actor sits on the edge of the bed. He does it the way a real person would,

bending at the waist, lap forming, hands falling to his sides. He is that good. He asks Marlene to think of someone she does not like, someone who maybe was mean to her, someone who was a friend but fell out.

"There was a girl named Amy — she was really sadistic..."

David S. looks at Marlene with the intensity of an actor who, with great training, also has been able to maintain a certain naturalness. "This Amy-bitch? Imagine if I were *her* inner voice instead. You would think it so unfair. Maybe this is the start of something good, because I'm here acting for you instead."

Marlene claims she doesn't know what to say.

"Line!" David S. calls out. "That's what we do, when an actor forgets his line. We call that out and someone feeds it to us and we go on. It's quite a cozy community." He starts to tuck his feet under the blankets until Marlene's face, wearing newly applied shades of appalled, speaks without saying a thing. "Ah, there are benefits to the dress rehearsal," he says. "Somebody would have told me this thing about the feet. They are the last place to circulate, you know."

"I don't love him anymore," Marlene blurts.

David S. is thrown from the bed.

"That is very good," he compliments. "Very well done. Who wrote that for you?" He walks around with the line in one hand. "Maybe that should be my line. As the inner voice, I should be telling you that." He moves his other hand over the air in the first hand, feeling each word. "I am so feeling that."

Encouraged, Marlene explains that while Alan is on top of her, she is restless. She tells the actor how she can't breathe sometimes and how they should have oxygen masks not just in planes but for the grounded too. She says they should have them in bedrooms, dining rooms at Thanksgiving, long grocery lines, and in school when the teacher is really boring.

"For these turbulent times we are not really living in," David S. says.

Marlene face-makes, which is like face painting but not as colorful or full of rainbows and unicorns. She tells the excellent actor that he's not helping.

"Help: to aid and abet," he says, walking around the bed, except for the part where the headboard is backed up against the wall. Inner voices cannot walk through things, after all. "What exactly is your contribution here? Look at you, which is hard to do, because there are no mirrors on the ceiling. Mirrors are a great tool for the actor. Expression is everything. So I'll tell you what I see—you're just there. It's like he's sexing it up with a corpse."

Marlene doesn't like being called dead.

"Well," David S. says, sitting cross-legged on the little throw rug near the night table on Marlene's side, "you are either dead or deadly. Other than the adverb ending tacked on, there's not much difference. But I know what alive is.

I know lively too. Actors, well, we are more alive than most. You, my dear, not even having a high school acting credit boasted about in the yearbook, well, you are rather, as the sheep say, 'blah.'"

"I take offense to that, sir," Marlene counters. "I am a pre-school teacher. And I know my animal sounds. And sheep go 'bah.'"

David S. uncrosses and stretches out, one leg at a time. "Blah. Bah. It's all the same. It depends where the lamp chops are from. Different parts of the country have different sheep accents. Ask any sheepologist. He'll tell you."

Marlene tries to maneuver a little beneath Alan's weight. She has changed her mind about David Strathairn the excellent actor. She tells him that she no longer likes him and his one-man show is over.

"You're telling me I'm kaput? It's too early for reviews," he says. "So you don't like me. Is it a momentary dislike or more of a pronounced one, like with Jim here?"

"His name is Alan. And please don't tell me that in certain parts of the country Alan is pronounced Jim and Jim is pronounced…"

"Natasha," David S. says.

After Marlene calls him insane, David S. tells her that she is ridiculous. "Look," he eloquently speaks, "call me insane; I don't care. I'd rather be insane—insanely handsome—insanely alive—insanely joyful. You see, ridiculous doesn't offer much in the way of living. It's kind of a joke on the person who is ridiculous." The actor places

his hand, it seems, gingerly on the side of the bed, and for Marlene, having had sesame ginger chicken with heartburn the evening before, well one can imagine her tentativeness with the whole thing. "You don't love him anymore. You've got to end this. Final credits running, you know? Even the longest running stage show closes. Movies get knocked off their #1 thrones all the time. Inevitability is a part of life that is hard for some, but inevitably, you have to accept that."

"Damn it," she says. "I don't want to hurt his feelings. He is a good person, just not my good person anymore."

David S. likes that Marlene used the word "damn." He thinks it's a good word. Meaningful. Expressive. Forceful. Alive. Damn. "You're not good together. You used to be. Something happened. Damn. Nobody ever tells you what happens after the 'and they lived happily ever after' part. Real life, you know, ruins everything. Did you know that the first year tulip bulbs come up, that's their best year of all? They're so straight and tall. But with each subsequent year they come back, they get shorter and shorter. Their beauty gets diminished slowly but certainly."

"I didn't know gardening was so depressing," Marlene muses. She tries body shifting slightly. The mattress creaks, "Get the hell off already."

"The pestilence is unbelievable," David S. says. He looks down at his pants, tracing a finger along the fabric. "How do they make these

things? Shh." He gets up to walk. His crossing thighs make that cutting swish sound corduroy makes. "The only article of clothing that gives a performance each time you wear it. I wonder if corduroy always has to be made in lines like this or if each leg can be just one big corduroy. Hey you—lady in bed—you're not sleeping on me, are you?"

Marlene opens her eyes. "No, no. I'm just reflecting," she says. "I reflect better with my eyes out."

The most excellent actor tsk-tsks her. "Let's check-list here. You're having sex with your boyfriend and you're bored out of your fucking mind. People jump off bridges all the time. People swim back to shore. People sink. Is this what you want for the rest of your life? Is it? Marlene, think. Before you answer. The clock is stripping. Ewwwww—time's up."

Marlene corrects him. "You mean ticking. The clock is ticking."

David S. corrects Marlene right back. "No. Stripping time where numbers tease us, scantily clad in their digital outlines, being peeled off, falling, falling, they've fallen and they can't get up. Hello, Marlene. This is life. This is your crappy life with a crappy sex life with a guy you no longer love. Oh, look's like the crap's won out."

Marlene had hoped for so much more. "I did, I really did," she says, blowing stray hairs out of her face. She wanted sex the way it is in the movies.

"Ah," David S. says, doing a happy dance. "Something I can relate to. Sex in the movies has writers, choreographers, directors, cinematographers, lighting designers, stunt doubles. And accountants. What is that look, Marlene? Yes, accountants. They make movie sex. It takes a whole payroll just to have the good sex."

Marlene has gotten extraordinarily comfortable with the actor in her bedroom while she is having crappy sex with her boyfriend. "You know," she says, "maybe this is just it for me."

David S. reaches deep inside fury. "You don't accept THIS. THIS is never IT. NEVER, do you hear?" He reaches inside comfort. He is that good an actor. It's like he's got one emotion in his front pocket and the other in the back. "After the break-up you'll get to eat a lot of ice cream in bed. And on the sofa. Watch a lot of sad movies. Some love stories. Wear those comfortable, totally non-gender specific pajamas you like so much. You'll have lots of empty picture frames once you take his out. Think of all the people possibilities you will be able to put in them."

Marlene inquiries about the possibilities, "I've always wanted to do a collage. Could I do a collage? And what about macaroni shell art? I always thought it never got its due beyond pre-school."

David S. tells Marlene that a good break-up eventually brings out the adventurer in a

person. "Once you lose all the weight you gain from all the ice cream. Then you can put on the adventurer clothes, and they will fit, and show off some cleavage. We may have to make you some though—cleavage, I mean." He adds that he doesn't really see the potential for pasta art, however he's been wrong before. "Tell him, Marlene. Tell him now."

And as Marlene begins to tell Alan that she needs him to stop, that they've got to talk, David Strathairn the excellent actor of so many movies like *Good Night and Good Light*, *The River Wild*, *L.A. Confidential*, and *The Bourne Ultimatum* and so many more, takes a bow. This leaves room for another excellent actor, Stephen Tobolowsky, to enter, confused at first, but then he looks down at the notes for his latest role: the inner voice for Alan. The notes say it's going to be a bad breakup, and so Stephen Tobolowsky gets to work, knowing that this will be different than the roles he had in *Groundhog Day*, *Thelma and Louise* and in *Glee*. He closes his eyes, breathes deep, and begins.

INTERVIEW: TODD LEVIN

WHAT HAVE YOU LOST THE MOST SLEEP OVER IN YOUR LIFE?

Todd Levin: As a comedy writer, I am constantly worried that, through some combination of age and contentment, the part of my brain that produces funny will shrivel up or peel away, and then I won't be able to work any longer and they'll repossess my flat screen television.

But here's a very real thought that once literally caused me to lose sleep for a very long time, when I was around 10 years old…I was just starting to think about the concept of death (as all good children do), and somehow I'd gotten it into my head that what if when we die we're still conscious of being dead? In other words, we're not buried alive—our bodies have expired, but there's still a spark of consciousness in our brain that is aware, just six feet above us, time keeps marching on. New things are being invented, the world is changing, etc. And our dead but conscious brain has to imagine all of it. That kept me up for nights, weeks, even months. And, on a few occasions, required waking up my parents for a second opinion.

DO YOU HAVE ANY ROUTINES OR REMEDIES FOR WHEN YOU CAN'T SLEEP?

Todd Levin: Read or masturbate. One of those tricks always works.

DO YOU HAVE ANY RECURRING DREAMS OR THEMES THAT POP UP REGULARLY?

Todd Levin: Not lately, really, although I used to regularly dream about my teeth falling out. It's a pretty common theme in dreams, I've been told, and it usually represents some fear of losing control. The teeth dreams were always my most vivid ones. I remember the feeling of trying to keep my teeth from falling out by gently biting down to hold them all in place, and feeling them rock back and forth in my gum beds. I can even remember, totally viscerally, the tiny clicks they made as they tumbled against each other when they fell out of my mouth, and the metallic taste of blood mixed with my saliva. Whenever I woke up from those dreams I was positive I was toothless.

These days the one theme I have noticed in my dreams is that I'm often trying (vainly) to convince other people I'm right/not crazy about something I'd either witnessed or heard, while other people in my dream are just flatly denying it. Had one of those dreams last night, actually.

HAVE YOU EVER SEEN CONAN O'BRIEN SLEEPING? IF SO, WAS IT ADORABLE OR AWKWARD OR SOMETHING ELSE?

Todd Levin: I've seen Conan resting, but I've never seen him sleep and I'm not totally convinced he does sleep. Conan is probably one of the most wired people I've ever been around, and in possession of one of the most active brains. I suppose his mind (and the minds of Joan Rivers, Steve Martin, Don Rickles, and Carl Reiner) are notable exceptions to my concern about losing funny.

SLEEPLESS IN SUBURBIA

MARY ROACH

Though I have always been a sound sleeper, I am frequently up at 4 a.m. This is around the time that my husband, Ed, having woken up at 3, will generally crawl back into bed. Ed goes downstairs to watch TV so that his tossing and turning doesn't wake me up.

This is very considerate, except that when he returns, he likes to chat about what he's been watching. The other night, Ed had been watching an infomercial for something called the Steam Shark. I have a distinct memory of surfacing from the depths of sleep directly into the sentence "You can steam-clean around the base of the toilet."

Last night it was "Honey, Bo Schembechler died."

Schembechler, Ed explained to my inert self, was a beloved University of Michigan football coach. There is little difference between talking to me about college football when I'm asleep and talking to me about it when I'm awake. Eyelid position, basically, is the difference. Ed kept going. "He was the voice of the Wolverines."

I was partly awake at this point, and for some reason, the sentence struck me as the funniest thing I'd heard in a very long time. Different rules apply between the hours of 2 and 4 a.m., I find. Things that would ordinarily not even qualify as mildly amusing will often, at 3 a.m., strike the ear as high comedy.

Worries are similarly warped.

I recently spent the hour from 4 to 5 a.m. worrying about the placement of two shrubs we had planted in our yard that day. Ed came in

from downstairs, and I unloaded my fears about the overly close positioning of the shrubbery. I made him promise that first thing the next day, we would dig one up and move it, lest they crowd each other's roots. In the morning, we went out to look at the plants. If anything, they looked a little lonesome there at 17 inches apart, just as the label had recommended. I am now known far and wide as the Nervous Gardener.

Anyway, once the laughter sets in, we're both up. The topic of wolverines led to savage animals in general, and, from there, to a game called African Veldt. We frequently make up mindless games to wile away the time until the sandman agrees to take over the proceedings again.

"First person to run out of animals is the loser," I said. Ed pointed out that since I had been to Africa, the game was rigged in my favor. He made me name three animals for every one of his.

"Fine. Leopard, zebra, elephant."

"Lion," said Ed with a great confidence.

"Warthog, wildebeest, springbok."

A long time went by. The shrubbery roots were closing in upon each other. Finally, and with great hesitancy, Ed said, "Giraffe?"

"Eland, gnu, ostrich."

"You can't do birds."

"Birds are animals."

"Okay, ant," said Ed, and then he rolled over. He took his bottom pillow and put it on top of his head. This is known as the Ed sandwich: pillow, Ed's head, pillow. He does this because he can't sleep if there's noise in the room. There isn't now, but there will be. I make noises while I sleep, and Ed has had many hours to devote to cataloging them. Common varietals include the Click, the Tommy Gun and the Darth Vader.

Light is also a problem for my husband. There can be no light in the bedroom, not even the light from the digital clock, which is hidden away on the bottom shelf of Ed's nightstand, broadcasting the time to toddlers and gnomes. The room across the hall must also be dark. We can't just close our bedroom door to block the light from that room, because this will make the bedroom too stuffy for Ed to sleep. That room must also have its curtains drawn. If he could, Ed would draw the curtains on the windows of our neighbors across the driveway, and on down the street, all the way to the horizon.

SNOWSTORM OF THE CENTURY

BILLY LOMBARDO

It was the year my father blamed a blizzard on me. It was cold that winter and a lot of snow. He had an old-school shovel—one of those big square-bladed jobs that curved at the top like a snowplow— heavy as hell—and you couldn't knock any sense into him

as about how the lighter ones were every bit as good.

"Every bit as good," he'd say, and then he'd roll his eyes and sigh long and disgusted, and blow out the letter *fffff*, like you were this close to making him swear.

Cold as it was that winter, on Groundhog Day it was fifty-six degrees; first time in a month above freezing. And sunny. I had forgotten about the sun.

How sunny it was was this. About two-thirty that day, I walked into my office after my last class and I bent over to pick up what I thought was a *post-it* note on the carpet. I even licked my finger and thumb so I could get a good grab at it. I bent over to pick it up, but when I got halfway down I saw that it was only a spot of sun bouncing off something shiny in the room. When I looked close and saw the rainbow-colored edges of the sunspot I sort of stayed bent over like that for a little while. My finger and my thumb were still ready to pinch at a piece of paper. Another teacher came in the office then and saw me bent over like that, and she asked me what was wrong. I told her nothing was wrong. I was just picking up a piece of paper. Then she

said, "Your phone's ringing. Why aren't you answering your phone?" and I told her I was just about to pick it up.

It was my father on the phone, complaining about the sump pump. It was working overtime with all the melting snow. He said it sounded like a river in the alley. There were rapids, he said, and a guy fishing in waders.

How I started the blizzard was this. I predicted we were done with snow for the year. What did I know? It was fifty-six that day. He just laughed and called me Tom Skilling. Tom Skilling is our weather guy.

And sure enough, a couple days later we got dumped with a foot of snow, heavy and wet. While we were shoveling he kept saying, "This blizzard is your fault, Skilling."

We went back in the kitchen for coffee after shoveling, and I was sitting at the table and he was sipping from his cup and standing—his back was too sore to sit. He pulled the tail of his tee shirt out of his pants and started rubbing his back—but not with his right hand like a normal person; he took the long way around with his left hand to make it seem like it was an impossible task for one man.

"I'm not gonna rub your back," I said. "I've been telling you to get rid of that—"

"Not the shovel again," he said.

He groaned and nodded at his back. "Come on," he said. "Five minutes."

"Trade shovels with me and I'll rub your back," I said.

"Never," he said.

"Rub it yourself, then," I said, and he stood there and kept trying to make the pain go away with the wrong hand.

"Next snowfall," he said. "We test the shovels. You and me. We'll set the shovels on the sidewalk and on the strength of their own downward weight we each shovel a line of snow and see who shovels a cleaner line."

"That test will prove nothing," I said.

"You're afraid," he said.

"No one shovels like that," I said.

"You're afraid," he said.

"Yeah, I'm afraid," I said.

"I knew it," he said.

"I'm not afraid," I said. "I was being facetious."

And he said, "Ohh, big word."

So just to shut him up, I said, "Fine. We'll do your stupid test," and before my coffee was finished he was on the carpet in the family room and I was rubbing his back, and it wasn't long before he started in about his back hairs.

His chest is totally bare except for six hairs that grow through a scar that runs the middle of his ribs. And on the other side, all he has are a few dozen crazy hairs on his lower back.

"How many of them back there?"

"I don't know," I said.

"Thirteen?"

"I don't know."

"Ballpark it," he said.

"I don't know, Dad."

"Jesus," he said. "All I'm asking is for a ballpark."

"Yeah," I said. "Thirteen."

"Do me a favor," he said.

"No."

"Come on," he said. "I'm not going another summer without taking my shirt off."

"You're seventy," I said. "You're not supposed to do that."

"Come on," he said.

"I'm barely forty, and I don't take my shirt off,"

"You never took your shirt off," he said.

"And trust me," I said, "if you take your shirt off, there'll be more to appall the neighbors than a couple dozen hairs on your back."

"A couple dozen?" he said. "I thought you said thirteen."

"I ballparked it," I said.

"Pull them out," he said. "Are they long enough to pull with your fingers?"

"I can pull them with my toes," I said.

"Your mother would have pulled them," he said. And then he said, "Forget it."

And that's what he was trying to do. He was trying to forget.

After a while he finally spoke again.

"Two-dozen?" he said.

"No, Dad. It's a dozen."

"Can you just count them?" he said.

And I stopped massaging.

"All right," he said. "You don't have to stop massaging."

"This isn't a massage," I said, and then he finally shut up. It sounded like the kitchen when the fridge stops humming. Sometimes you forget about the quiet.

★ ★ ★

My old man swears by peanut oil and its healing properties. There's a bottle of it in the nightstand by his bed. The drawer is darkened with oil stains. How many times I had seen my mother standing over him, warming oil in her hands before rubbing it on his back or thumbing it in the purple scar on his chest.

After a while he reached his hand, sleepily, out to the side. I think he thought he was on his bed and he was reaching for the oil, and so I whispered, "I'll be right back," and I got the peanut oil.

I warmed it up so I wouldn't have to hear about how cold it was, and pretty soon he started groaning again.

"Mmgh," he said. "Right there."

I kept going at that spot, trying to get at whatever knot was there and then he said, "Oh, right there, honey," and I knew he was thinking about mom.

Then he said, "Goddamn snow," but it wasn't the snow he was damning.

Pretty soon his breathing deepened, and so I figured I'd stop, and I reached for his tee shirt with my right hand while I kept at his back with my left; I figured I'd fade away from the massage slowly so as not to wake him, but when I looked at my hand against his yellowing tee shirt I noticed I had rubbed out a couple of those long hairs. They

were peanut oiled to my hand. I looked at them for a minute. I was almost laughing, I think. And then I put the tee shirt on the carpet and started massaging him again. I figured I'd just keep going at him until all of the hairs came out.

★ ★ ★

That wasn't the last we saw of the snow that winter. On Valentine's Day we got socked again. They actually called it a blizzard and closed the school for two days and while all the students were sledding at the landfill they turned into a toboggan run, I spent the snow days at my father's house. On the news they were calling it *The Snowstorm of the Century*.

At about nine o'clock that first night we went through with the test of the shovels. At first I was a little grumpy about it because it was a stupid test, but as soon as I set the edge of my shovel down I was all of a sudden excited. I felt the potential of my shovel; I felt its capacity. I envisioned the clean scrape of it from the bottom stair of the front porch to the end of the property line. But my father said, "One, two, three, go!" and he quickstarted me, like it was a race we were having and not just a shovel test, and I could see the blade of his shovel—which had been rusting into an upward curl for years—it wasn't catching the lowest layer of snow, but I could see from the excitement in his back and in his arms that he felt he had the test in the bag.

And just about then is when my shovel slammed into a crack in the sidewalk, and though it was snowing too much for me to hear him, I could see from his head that he was laughing. Head thrown back and the streetlight there, and the snow coming down. And I knew it would serve no purpose to explain to him what was holding me up, so I just started laughing, too.

I lowered the handle of my shovel to raise the blade off the walk, and now it slid atop the snow like a sled. I wanted him to turn around and see my lesser path. I wanted him to keep laughing. I couldn't remember the last time he looked so happy. He pumped his arm and held his finger in the air like that beast was the number one shovel in the world.

And then we cleared the walk. We cleared the station wagon. We shoveled the stairs and the gangway out to the alley and the neighbors' sidewalks and a parking place for the old lady down the street. We cleared away everything.

All that Valentine's Day they kept interrupting the news to cut back to Tom Skilling for an update, and you could tell they were forcing him to use that phrase, *Snowstorm of the Century*. You could just tell. He was sort of overdoing it. He would do this thing with his voice—he would make almost like he was an actor on a stage—and this thing with his fist, too; he would sort of pump it across his chest. It was like they wanted us to think it was up to Tom Skilling to get us through the blizzard. But all he wanted to do was give you

the necessary information on the storm system. He wanted you to know *why* it was storming, *why* there was a blizzard, and he wanted you to know when everything was going to be back to normal again.

It was my father, a couple of weeks before, who had told me the story about Tom Skilling's brother and that mess he'd gotten into with Enron. I never paid too much attention to all that, but the old man was all over it. He's how I found out about Skilling's brother going to prison. And my old man could tell it was killing Tom. He could see it in his eyes.

"Stuff like that *consumes* a man," my father said, and then he looked at me like he was pretty sure I'd be happy he used a word like that. And then he said it again.

"It just *consumes*. Maybe you forget about it every once in a while, but then it hits you all of a sudden like a punch in the belly, and then you think you'll never forget it again. Like it will be impossible to forget."

And then my father shook his head at the torments of men.

During the commercial I went into the kitchen to get a couple of cookies for our cocoa, and when I returned to the family room Skilling was just about to turn the cameras over to the anchors. My dad dunked his cookie into his hot chocolate and held it over his cup to let it drip, and I know me and my dad were thinking the same thing, because my dad said, "Look. Look at him. They want him to say it again."

And he said, "Don't do it, Tom. Don't say it. That ain't the Snowstorm of the Century, Tom. That ain't even a storm. I'll—I'll tell you about a storm." And then he looked at me and said, "How about it, kiddo. You and me—you and me could tell him about storms."

And just then Skilling looked at me and my dad sitting on the couch in the living room, and he made this face I can't get out of my head. He pressed his lips together into a forced smile and he nodded his head and looked at us, and he said, "Look, guys. I'm sorry. Some things. Some things are bigger than snow. There's some things you can't just put a shovel to."

PHILOSOPHY / SCIENCE OF NATURE / MATHEMATICS / MIXED / ACOUSTICS OR, THE BED FRAME

JAMES TADD ADCOX

My girlfriend has been depressed most of the winter. She claims that this is because our bed frame creaks. In fairness to my girlfriend, creaks is too gentle a word for what this

bed frame does. Every time one or the other of us makes the slightest movement in bed, the bed frame makes a noise like a pair of ancient automobiles coupling. It's difficult to get through an entire night without being woken up once or twice. I don't even bother bringing sex up anymore.

My girlfriend has a theory, involving sound waves and how certain frequencies interact with the brain, that she says establishes a direct correspondence between our bed frame and her depression. She shared this theory with me for the first time earlier today. I didn't point out that, in fact, she was depressed for several months before the bed frame began creaking. "So fine," I say. "Let's buy another bed frame." I'm in the living room, trying to figure out what to put in column 11b of a tax form. Do I even need to fill in column 11b? Am I supposed to initial somewhere nearby?

"Can't," my girlfriend says. She's in the bedroom, from the sound of things examining the bed frame. "We don't have the sort of money to be splurging on bed frames. And it's only this one part that creaks."

"So let's throw out that part." There's a long silence that I take to mean that what I just said was somehow idiotic.

"That part connects to this other part, which is the crossbar," she says. "There's no taking out that part." She decides the best course of action is to layer tape over that part, to muffle the sound, maybe. She's in there for a while. There's more noise involved than one would expect.

"How's it going?" I call out.

"I'm still sad," she calls back.

"Is the bed frame fixed?"

"I took the bed frame apart. We can sleep on the mattress."

"Are you sure you shouldn't see a counselor or something?" I ask.

"I'm seeing one," she says. "Her name is Mandy."

"You've told me that before," I say, biting the end of my pen.

"I've told you that before," she says.

INLAID OLIVE TREES

CATRIONA WRIGHT

"Dad, I can do it," Kate protests. "Thanks for all your help and everything, but you can go now."

The firmness of her tone strikes me as both condescending and deluded.

"Don't be ridiculous," I say. "Pass me that screwdriver."

Kate appraises me like I'm a huge puddle of water and she's trying to decide whether she can leap over and still remain dry.

"*Pretty please* pass me the screwdriver," I say. Yanked from her mental risk assessment, she smiles and hands it to me headfirst. Both of us hold it for a moment before she releases her grip.

There's no way in hell Kate would be able to assemble this bed herself. She would have a tough time putting together a Kinder Surprise toy, let alone a bed. At least she was wise enough to avoid another packed sawdust and fiddly bits Ikea contraption. She sold her white ASPELUND—which *I* assembled.

The bed I carried in today, piece by clunking piece, is sturdy, made of thick oak boards, stained to amber. Scratched, aged, it is the bed Andrea and I slept in and romped around on before the divorce.

Three weeks ago it was delivered by Andrea's new husband, Edward, not to this new place on Grace, but to the old Annex apartment.

"Couldn't Prince Charming have waited to drop it off here?" I'd said as I sweated up the stairs with the mattress.

Kate had lowered her chin and rubbed the back of her neck. "I didn't ask," she'd mumbled, glancing at me from the top of her eyes.

Sometimes I find it hard to tell whether Kate respects Edward or thinks he's full of shit. Maybe it's just because I'm the ex-husband, but I think the guy's full of shit, what with his ironed jeans and debonair politeness, the pretentious way he kisses Andrea on the tip of her nose when he says goodbye, his thick—blatantly plucked—eyebrows.

★ ★ ★

Without bothering to organize all of the bed's components—crosspieces, legs, strapped roll of slats—I pick up the footboard and grab a screw. How hard can it be? I'm sure I can figure it out as I go along.

As I work, I become aware of my heartbeat. It amplifies through the apartment, bounces off the cream walls and wooden-shuttered bay window. Three years ago I was diagnosed with hypertension and angina. My doctor put me on Adalat and forbade me from eating grapefruit. Something about increasing or decreasing the effect of the drugs. For weeks all I could dream about was pink grapefruit, segmented, sugared, the perfect balance of tart and sweet. In the grocery store I would gaze at the mounds of rough yellow orbs as if they were all the blowjobs I was no longer getting. In truth, I don't care much for grapefruit. I just loathe the idea that pharmaceutical whims are allowed to dictate my choices. Mercifully, that aspect of my life is now under control. In addition to taking Adalat, I carry around nitroglycerin pills.

★ ★ ★

One afternoon when Kate was seven years old, Andrea accompanied her to an afternoon piano lesson with Miss Beard. Their homecoming sent cold air gusting through the living room. The front door clanged shut. I could hear them stamping their boots.

"How's my little Mozart?" I yelled. Rising from my armchair, I toppled a half-empty bottle of beer, but grabbed it by the neck before losing any. Nobody answered. I went out into the front hallway, feeling tipsy and content.

"How's my little…" I repeated, but stopped, abashed, when I saw the plaintive expressions on their faces.

"Sure you aren't mad?" Kate whined, peering up at Andrea.

"I'm sure," Andrea said wearily, unwinding Kate's scarf from her neck. The zipper on Kate's coat got stuck halfway, so Andrea had to zip it all the way up before trying again.

"What if I promise to practice every single day? Will that make up for it?"

The zipper cooperated. Andrea hung Kate's coat on the wall and began taking off her own. "You didn't do anything wrong, honey."

"I'm sorry I keep asking. I'm sorry. Am I annoying you? You aren't mad that I keep asking?"

Andrea crouched down to Kate's height. "Why don't I make you a peanut butter and banana sandwich?"

"My tummy hurts," Kate said. "Is it okay if I go to my room?"

"Whatever you want." Andrea waved at me and smiled wanly.

Snow had drifted off them and begun to melt on the brown tiles.

"Daddy," Kate came over and hugged me. With my beer-free hand, I hugged back. Through my shirt, I could feel her cold body. She headed to her room.

Andrea indicated that I should follow her into the kitchen. We shut the door.

"What was that all about?" I said.

"Another student arrived late for his lesson and Kate didn't want him to hear her. It threw her right off. She got really agitated. Miss Beard managed to calm her down, but when she started playing 'Ode to Joy' she kept getting stuck on the third bar. Every time she made a mistake, she would insist on starting over. The first three bars, again and again. She was getting red in the face—"

"But she plays that song all the time," I interrupted.

Andrea's eyes flared. "Not in front of an audience she doesn't. She got so upset she started to dry heave. Honestly, I thought she was going to vomit! We had to stop the lesson."

"Poor kid," I said. "I remember how nervous I used to get before clarinet recitals."

Andrea paced from the stove to the backdoor. "It's not normal to be *that* worried." With a squelch, she sat on a stool behind the counter. "I think we should take her to see someone."

"No need to blow it out of proportion." I put down my beer and massaged her shoulder. "It's just a bit of performance anxiety. She'll grow out of it."

But she didn't.

Kate's anxiety worsened. Worries began to stick to her mind like burrs. She worried about spelling tests and acid rain. She repeatedly asked if Andrea and I were going to get a divorce. I installed a night-light in her bedroom. She was nervous about the homeless man outside the grocery store; his coat thin as the paper bags we carried to the car. Andrea and I never talked about wars or natural disasters or credit card bills in front of her. Andrea was careful about which movies we let her watch. Kate was convinced that she would get leukemia and all her hair would fall out. She wanted to know exactly how to get to heaven. Whenever we left the house, she would twist the door handle four times, just to quadruple-check that it was locked.

★ ★ ★

"Can I help with anything?" Kate says. "Or do you mind if I just start unpacking the rest of my stuff?"

"Unpack away," I say. At this point I've helped Kate move so many times we've streamlined the operation down to two hours, and that includes

U-Haul rental and return. It's the unpacking that takes forever. Kate will rearrange her furniture over and over again like a cat kneading a lap before it will condescend to lie down.

"Wait," Kate says, "are you really supposed to be screwing there? It looks like you're splintering the wood or warping it a bit. See, right there."

"I know what I'm doing," I say. "Go on. Unpack your heart out."

"I don't have to do it right this second. The screw is just a bit. Watch out, you're forcing it, you're going to…"

I put the screwdriver down and glare at her.

"Okay," she relents. "Okay. Positive you don't want anything? Seriously, Dad, you're breathing kind of hard. Want me to get you some water or juice? An apple?"

"You know what," I say, "you could go and buy me a coffee." This way, I think, I can get rid of her for a couple minutes, and figure out how to put this damn thing back together properly. She's right about the screw; I'm splintering the wood.

"Do you want me to?" she says. "Is that what you want?"

"For Christ's sake, Kate. Yes. Yes."
She looks down.

"Sorry," I say, gently, "I didn't mean to yell, it's just that…"

"I know," she says. "Do you want milk and sugar? What if they only have cream? Is cream okay?"

"Cream is fine."

She's your daughter, I tell myself, it's not her fault, it's not your fault, it's not Andrea's fault, it's not anybody's fault. It's just the way she is.

★ ★ ★

Kate was conceived in this bed. It was a wedding present from Andrea's Uncle Wayne, a widowed farmer and amateur carpenter, who dropped it off at our new house in his pickup truck. When we got it upstairs, we noticed sun-bleached cornhusks stuck like toilet paper to the legs. I started to tear them off, but Andrea insisted we leave them. As for Wayne, he got around to putting it together. He assembled it all himself, wouldn't even let us help.

When he was done, he threw us a good-natured smirk. "Guaranteed to hold up under any strain," he said, "or your money back."

A generous Queen with high, thick legs and an arched headboard, plain except for two olive trees carved into the corners, the bed took up most of the master bedroom.

At first Andrea and I made little use of the bed's size—at least, for sleep. We would doze off entwined in the middle. We even had to flip the mattress to flatten the resultant trough. But after Kate was born, Andrea began to insist that she couldn't fall asleep if we were touching. Not even an elbow or pinkie toe. After sex she would peck me on the lips and scoot to her side of the bed: a maneuver I nicknamed the *un*screw. Although, rationally, I understood why Andrea

needed a good night's rest—Katie was a difficult baby and I wasn't much help with my late office hours, and, besides, aren't men supposed to hate cuddling?—it was still hard not to feel that her body was denying mine.

Part of me was hoping that Andrea would be here today. This morning, however, my daughter informed me that her mother had to be at work. I suspect this is a lie. Andrea is a greeting-card designer and makes her own hours. She's probably still pissed about the fact that my cell phone went off in the middle of her wedding ceremony to Edward. It's not that I have any aspirations of getting back together with Andrea. I just like the occasional run-in... they affirm that I was once capable of sustaining the staring contest of marriage.

Recently, I've begun making tentative forays into Internet dating. My profile is sparse, pictureless, a non-committal "just looking" rather than a naked and (I can't help feeling) pathetic admission that I'm in the market for a "long-term relationship." I haven't disclosed my new amorous habits to anyone. I'm still working out my spin on it. Self-deprecatory admission about the difficulty of finding a mate when you're deep in your fifties and in possession of a paunch? Defensive—and a touch self-aggrandizing— excuses about my busy, busy, important life and my utter lack of disposable time? The fact is, I'm not sure yet what *I* think about the whole set-up. Whether I should feel exhilarated, depressed or embarrassed when I scroll down the pages

and pages of women with their coy or hopeful expressions, their interests veering from "flying trapeze" to "watching television." Whenever I decide to actually write a come-hither (scrambling my voice with Microsoft Thesaurus) I'm convulsed with doubt. Is it even possible to force Cupid's hand in this way?

★ ★ ★

"I brought milk and cream," Kate says as she walks into the room. "Looks like you're making good progress."

In truth, I've barely done anything since she left.

"Milk, please," I say.

She reaches into her pocket and extracts a small milk container. She hands it to me along with the Styrofoam cup.

Steam rises around my mouth as I sip.

"I'll just be over here, unpacking" she says. "Yell if you need anything." The entire apartment is only four hundred and fifty square feet. I could whisper and she would hear.

★ ★ ★

Kate had trouble sleeping when she was a kid. Nightmares would propel her to our bed. Her breath steadying between us, further unsteadying us. It was petty, but I hated that Andrea slept peacefully on these nights, didn't mind being kicked and punched by Kate, didn't

mind her daughter's hot breath on her neck. By the time Kate turned twelve, I was often sleeping on the couch. The first couch-bound sleep occurred the night after I found out that Andrea had taken Kate to a shrink without telling me. I had discovered the bottle of anti-anxiety medication on the table in the front hall. When Andrea returned from grocery shopping, I maraca-rattled the pills in her face.

"What is this about?"

She placed a milk carton in the door of the refrigerator. "The doctor thinks it'll help."

"I don't want my daughter to be part of the overmedicated generation."

She closed the door. "This isn't about what you want."

★ ★ ★

Rejuvenated by coffee, I tackle the bed-frame again. I screw the footboard to the sidepieces. Flushed, I stop for a minute. Once my pulse settles, I haul the headboard off the ground. Right as I'm about to rotate a screw in, I notice that the two olive carvings are facing out. I glance over at my daughter. She's unwrapping mugs from newspaper and humming some pop song. Relieved that she didn't notice, it takes me a moment to recognize the mugs. Heavy mugs, glazed with a green that bleeds from forest at the rim to lime at the base, the thick handles curved into half-hearts, they were wedding presents, too. Andrea must have given them to Kate along

with the bed. The weight of the headboard becomes daunting. It crashes to the floor, sending screws jangling across the hardwood. Startled, Kate turns. I blink and wave my hand dismissively. To avoid her concerned expression, I lean down, and run my fingers over the raised olive trees before I lift the board. Again.

★ ★ ★

Around the time that I was spending most nights on the couch, Kate's night terrors morphed into insomnia. Once or twice a month, and with increasing frequency, she wouldn't sleep at all. Her wakefulness gave us our first true daughter-father tradition. At some point past midnight, she would lope downstairs and I would put a pan of milk on the stove, boil it until its surface thickened to puckered leather, pour it out into two mugs. Add a teaspoon of honey to hers. A couple shots of whiskey to mine. We would sit together in the living room. Kate would recline on the couch, pillows and blankets heaped around her in the hopes that they could pull her into dreams. I would sit sentinel in a nearby chair; with my free hand, I would brush the velvet armrest, watching the fabric lighten on the upstroke and darken on the down. While we sipped our drinks, we would listen to the *Goldberg Variations*.

Although I knew I should be happy when I didn't hear Kate's soft footsteps on the stairs, I couldn't help but feel a bit disappointed. I

enjoyed our late nights together. The two of us listening to Glenn Gould's hands skipping across the keys. Often when I'm bewildered or sad, I will repeat that familiar routine for myself. Whiskey, milk, Bach.

If Kate dozed off on the couch, I had no choice but to crawl back into bed with Andrea, careful to keep a distance between us, yet renewed by the feeling that I had helped Kate.

"What're you doing here?" Andrea would mumble.

"Kate's downstairs."

Hearing this, she would loosen some covers and toss them to my side.

I would fall asleep thinking that nothing was unfixable.

★ ★ ★

"You haven't said anything about the place yet," Kate says, "do you like it?"

"Much better than your last place," I say. "Definitely an upgrade."

"You always say that," Kate says.

"This time, I mean it," I say. "It's a great bachlorette pad. High ceilings, new appliances, wood floors, no mouse shit chocolate-sprinkled in the cupboards. You won't even notice the tilted floorboards after a while."

Kate smiles. "How's it going there?"

"Almost," I say, "I'll need your help in a sec."

All that remains to be done is to attach the centre support rail, lay down the slats, and heave the mattress on. Kate walks over to me and watches, silent, as I work. We each unroll a section of slats, making sure they align together.

★ ★ ★

I can still be startled by my daughter—her suddenly grown-up face; her cheeks, free of baby fat; her thin blond hair cut into a short stylish bob that makes it look full, healthy. Dry skin peels on her nose, but no acne mottles her forehead. Today she is wearing a bright blue cardigan and small rose earrings.

At fourteen, Kate looked far different. Chubby, fond of black eyeliner and white nail polish, her hair a seaweed-straggle of knots. She wore shapeless black sweatshirts and baggy jeans, hoop earrings big enough to be bracelets, clunking Doc Martens.

"A phase," I said, even after I glimpsed Kate's arms covered in deep scratches, congealing into scabs. I had chosen to interpret my wife's concerns as accusations against me—my long work hours and affection for single malt. "You heard her," I said. "She gets itchy. She scratches in her sleep."

"You actually believe that?"

"I trust her," I said, self-righteously, untruthfully.

★ ★ ★

After Kate's suicide attempt—a bottle of Tylenol, all her anxiety meds, a mug of my

whiskey—she was admitted to the hospital for two weeks. During that time Andrea and I slept in the bed, together again. Neither of us had to ask. Not only were we in the same bed, it was like before Kate was born: my arms snug around her, our legs braided together, Andrea's head on my collarbone, ear pressed against the thickening thump of my heart.

★ ★ ★

Together, Kate and I lift the mattress onto the bed. Afterwards I raise my hand to my chest, hoping to coax out the tension gathering there. Kate seems like she is about to say something but stops herself; instead, she falls back, star-fished, onto the mattress. I still can't figure out how to feel about her body, dreaming, vulnerable, on the ex-marital bed. Even more jarring is the thought of Kate having sex on it. The thought that, if a hyper-sensitive lithograph were made of the mattress, then on the print, Kate's body would be indistinguishable from Andrea's or mine—worse, it would be indistinguishable from Edward's, or from Kate's inferred lover. Time compressed, leveled, our bodies all making promises to each other. But I'm getting ahead of myself. As far as I know she doesn't have a boyfriend or girlfriend. Last April I did notice a pack of birth control pills in her bathroom.

And there was once a boy named Matt or Brendan, but that was years ago. Generally, I avoid asking about those kinds of things.

Kate sits up.

"I've always loved this bed" she says, "especially these inlaid olive trees. Do you think they're an allusion to the *Odyssey*?"

After three false starts—nursing, cooking and business—Kate at last seems to have settled into a classics B.A. at the University of Toronto. Not the most lucrative choice ever, but what can you do?

"Maybe," I say. Wait, have I even *read* the *Odyssey*? "Remind me of that part again."

She speaks in a tone new to her repertoire, a quick confident flow:

"It's the final test Penelope gives Odysseus to be totally positive that it's really him: her husband who has been gone for twenty years. Penelope asks the servant to move the bed, but Odysseus protests because he made the bed himself and so he knows that one of the legs is a living olive tree. It's the moment when Penelope looks at Odysseus and Odysseus looks at Penelope and they're lost in mutual revelation. The revelation of their absolute like-mindedness."

For an instant I think she's talking about Andrea and me. The story feels like an interrogation light, scorching my eyes, setting my heart to stagger. But this paranoia retreats as I search my daughter's relaxed, almost self-satisfied, face. She's just showing off.

"Somehow I doubt that Uncle Wayne was aware of the connection," I say, "but it's a nice story."

"Luckily, we can move *this* bed." She laughs. "Where do you think it should go?"

"Do we have to move it? It looks fine here."

"What about over there?" Kate points to the other side of the room. "Do you want to at least see? I mean you don't have to, I can probably—"

"Sure. Fine. Whatever."

Straining, we shuffle the bed to the other side of the room. Sweat dribbles down my forehead.

Kate takes several steps back and appraises the new arrangement. "You were right. It looked better over there." She lifts her side.

"Just give me a minute," I say. "My arm hurts a bit."

She lowers the bed and approaches me. Unlike Odysseus I probably would have ordered the servant to move the damn thing. Aches shudder across my neck and shoulders. Out of forgetfulness or stubbornness or utter self-absorption I would have lost the girl, everything. My chest tightens. Without even realizing the scope of my mistake. I slump on the bed. Kate sits beside me, rubbing my back.

"Dad," she says in a firm voice. "Where're your pills?"

"In my bag," I wheeze. She strides toward the other side of the room and shakes a pill from the bottle. She offers it to me. My daughter, my grown daughter, my kind and wise daughter and suddenly competent daughter, offers it to me.

"Lie down," she says, putting her hand on my shoulder.

"I'm fine."

"Just for a second." She pushes me down with stubborn gentleness. "I'll be right here."

I yield to her, lying back on the bed.

As the pill dissolves beneath my tongue into a sting and bitter taste, I think once again about grapefruits.

★ ★ ★

The first morning after Kate came back from the hospital, Andrea and I woke early to make blueberry pancakes with whip cream. Andrea kept them warm on the stove, letting Kate sleep in until one. While we waited, we drank two pots of coffee. When Kate emerged and sat down at the kitchen table, we both asked her how she had slept.

"Jinks," I said to Andrea, "you owe me a coke."

Andrea laughed with forced boisterousness. Kate smiled with the left side of her mouth.

"Fine," Kate said, "considering."

"Want some pancakes?" Andrea said, hopefully.

Kate sat with her shoulders hunched. The expression in her eyes was unstable, straining toward remoteness like a hand held over a mouth, attempting to silence some confession: embarrassment, remorse. Perhaps

disappointment. "I'm not really that hungry," she murmured.

"Honey, you have to have something," Andrea said. "What about grapefruit?"

"I guess that would be okay."

"Count me in!" I said.

Andrea cleaved two fruits in half. The insides were a blanched pink. Using a small, sharp knife, she scored them into wedges. She presented them to us in blue bowls.

"Voilà," Andrea said.

The grapefruit was fibrous, acidic. All wrong.

Wordlessly, Kate rose from the table and got the sugar from its post beside the stove. We accepted this solution, pouring crystals on until they formed a thin frost.

HANDS TO WORK

STEVE HIMMER

In the hours between *Girls Gone Wild* ads over and over and the modestly hot weather women of early news, skip across stations and alight on aged actresses you once dreamt about, now selling blenders and treadmills. Listen too long as has-been *Playboy* bunnies explain herbal home

cures and real estate schemes, how to get rich and get bigger and satisfy woman and wallet. Sit near the screen with the volume way down because six years of wife and three months of daughter are sleeping a ceiling away.

"Not tonight," she snapped at your hand creeping up on her thigh. "Not yet," and so back downstairs, back to the nighttime TV that stands in for insomniacs' dreams. She's worn out from hourly feedings and still recovering under the surface. Her body a mystery for the first time since college when you noticed the girl down the hall, but this time you can't read the clues. This time you can't crack the case.

You decided together to distend the circle of being a couple and become a triangle instead, to add those sharp edges to your life together, and she pulled you atop her four and five times a day on the couch, on the floor, even in the back of the car. It was dorm room passion all over again, and you secretly hoped it would take her awhile. You looked forward to a few months of trying, of testing positions and styles, but she was pregnant as soon as you tried. As soon as you agreed to start trying. And now there's the baby, perfect and powerful and terrifying, the rest of your life all wrapped up in a diaper too big for her body but too small to contain everything that flows

from it. They sleep with their noses together and breathing in sync, knees pulled up into a perfect heart shape, and outside it you are the unpiercing arrow who watches TV in the dark.

Your bleary eyes catch on a long, shapely leg but flesh turns to ash as you watch Shakers turn tables and chairs on pre-dawn PBS. Startled by the deceit, you linger and learn how unwelcome desires become other urges, how the crackling electricity of lust powers bandsaws and routers, spins spindles out by the cartload and keeps Brothers from thinking about other legs of softer substance and only a long hall away—women at one end of the building and men at the other, with enough of a walk in between for a body to forget why it started out walking before it arrives, before getting itself into trouble. Every rug woven and each sweater spread taut between needles is a thick curtain drawn across curious eyes, drawn between bodies and souls. Every tabletop sanded smooth is a shield, to keep crafty hands from idling.

Your hands worked some wood back in high school when everyone had to—all the boys, anyway, in those days when girls were still different and delicate and expended their energies on home economics—but not after marriage offered other ways to spend time. You moved here with only a hammer and saw, both of them rusty and one of them dull, hardly enough to fix what might break in a home. But there are the tools of the man who sold you this house, better tools, bigger: a drill press and lathe, a router and planer and machines you can't name but could smooth wood or mangle a limb as easily as they turn on. He threw in the tools not to sweeten the deal or because you asked for them, but he saw no time for woodwork with so many widows in his new retirement village. He winked when he tossed you that detail.

Now in the smallest of hours, two stories away from your daughter and wife, pull a blank of pale wood from the stack by the lathe and set the motor to turning. Unroll chisels kept safe in their soft sheepskin sleeves and press a round blade to the rotating grain. Try to remember what little your hands once knew about wood. Ease the tip, move it slowly, anticipate the bite and first feathered blonde curl. No more TV, no more awkward advances and mumbled regrets. Instead cradles and tables to fill up the house, a new bed to sleep in each night forever if that's what it takes. Forests will fall to the honed teeth and blades of your recast desire, soft white wood giving way to a chisel's steel gleam.

But the blade is too dull or the touch is too rushed. Instead of smooth shaving you gouge out a chunk and the blank—not so secure in its mount as it seemed—unmoors from the lathe and kicks into the air, rams your chin so your teeth clamp your tongue and you see nothing but stars though it's almost sunrise outside. The chisel blade bites a half-moon from your palm, leaving a thick flap of flesh and a fast flow of blood.

The first red streak of morning finds you in the cellar, red-handed on a rickety stool.

Squeeze one hand with the other, but that's not enough to stop yourself spilling all over the floor. Wrap the wound up in one of your socks from a pile of laundry that's waited a long time for washing. Creep upstairs in hope of getting into the bathroom and cleaning yourself without leaving a trail through the kitchen.

Shove your stained pajama bottoms down deep in the hamper and try to slide into bed without waking your wife or the baby between your two bodies. Slide under the blankets as if you've been there beside them all night, and wrap your throbbing arm around as much as you can and think about where all the Shakers have gone.

RIDING THE BUS

RACHEL MANS

Leda was half-Greek, her father's side. She told Hector when he'd proposed, that no arguments, that she was hyphenating their last name. "Greeks are the god-makers," she'd told him. "It's worth a few extra syllables." Another sacrifice made to Zeus, this one by a nice Christian girl.

She'd kissed him good night outside of the restaurant, said 'Be good' and laughed. Hector met Joey in the parking lot after dinner; they'd dressed up for this pizza place like it was some kind of trial run of the rehearsal dinner tomorrow. The two of them shot-gunned beers in the back of the Joey's van. They drove through the dark, suburban landscape of Eagan and ended up on a patch of dewy grass somewhere in a neighborhood roundabout. Hector lay flat on the grass and Joey sprawled next to him.

Hector's head was spinning and the dew felt like sweat on the back of his dress shirt. "Take me somewhere," Hector said. Why did he wear a dress shirt? "I don't care where. Get me a bed." He felt his mind slowing, a tunnel approaching.

"You feeling okay?" Joey asked.

"I'm feeling tall. I don't know. How should I feel?"

"Tall's just fine. Tall's great," Joey said.

Hector wondered if you could get grass stains on your skin. He thought about Leda, his bride. His girl, Leda. She'd be asleep by now at her parents'.

"Joey," he said, "I'm going to break Leda."

"You couldn't hurt a dog that was biting you, man," was Joey's response, and he passed him a flask.

Hector unscrewed the lid and took a pull. "She's going to fall apart when she marries me."

"Trust me. Marriage is marriage is marriage. She's dealt with you this long."

Hector looked up at the sky and saw streetlamps that looked like a row of moons. She'd be broken down. Maybe it wouldn't be soon, but sometime. Maybe fifty years from now. Just when she felt safe, after two generations were firmly popped out with their blended genes, she'd see that something terrible in him, or maybe she'd seen it all along and it finally would overwhelm all the good in her one day. "I am not a good man," Hector said to the moons and to Joey, and he threw up on the grass, the tree root under his head, and himself.

In the morning, his internal clock tried to right itself. It felt like eight-thirty, give or take. He'd always had a good sense of time. A few thoughts occurred to Hector. Thought number one came paired with a headache: too much whiskey. Thought number two immediately followed with a rush of nausea: never that much whiskey again.

His senses had shut themselves off out of necessity, but they returned with the pain in his head. The air smelled like peonies. He opened his eyes. He was in bed. I'm in bed, he thought.

In a bed, that is, not his. Not Leda's either. With the crispness of the sheets, he knew it must have been a motel. It was a nice bed though, and he was picky about beds.

But the weight of waking up in a strange motel room fell upon his chest suddenly, and as

that thought processed, a little dam of nausea burst.

"Oh, God," he said.

"He'll forgive you," a voice answered. "So will I, and I'm sure the maid staff's dealt with worse."

A fat voice. His mother's. He raised himself up on his elbows. His mother sat on the chair in the corner of the motel room, a newspaper in front of her face like a curtain.

She lowered it and looked at him with those same thin eyebrows he had, and dirt-brown eyes. "I'm supposed to tell you that Joey would've taken you back with him, but that his wife was already going to be mad enough about his drunk ass showing up. Bachelor parties. I swear." She unperched herself from the chair and sat on the bed's edge. Her wide hips made a curving imprint in the mattress. "He found my motel number on a piece of paper in your pocket. You're lucky I love you, dragging your drunk corpse into the sheets like that."

"I didn't know where I was."

"I hope you're not used to motel rooms, kiddo." She stood up and adjusted a vase of fresh flowers on the table. There. Peonies. His mother always half-moved into hotel rooms while she was in them. Quilts, flowers. He made a sound as she touched them, and she said, "I got these from your aunt's yard. You could visit her. She's up in St. Paul now, you know."

"I will. We will," he said. "Me and Leda."

They were going to have four kids, he and Leda. He thought about them as he rode in the

Number Six bus back to his apartment. His relatives, staying in the same motel, had supplied him with something clean to wear, more than happy to give the future groom clothes. No one likes a naked groom, they joked. Not even the bride! Hilarious. The clothes itched. Eleven-thirty now, he knew, with his watch back on. Four kids. If he had his way, it'd be three boys and a girl, but Leda wanted twin girls. Leda'd look good pregnant. She was wirey, and he found it attractive when thin women got pregnant, carrying the baby like a shoplifted watermelon under a skinny kid's shirt. He got that image from a comic one time. The shop owner in the comic had said, "They get younger and younger."

Leda.

In his law school days, when she was a hundred miles away, he'd call her every night and just so they could breathe at each other. With nothing to say and no reason to hang up, no good reason besides more Torts or Property, he'd just breathe. He felt like he hadn't taken a breath until he was on the phone with her. Sometimes he'd tell her jokes out of a joke book they'd gotten from a thrift store. She'd laugh, but the phone would pick it up as static. Better to just breathe.

Leda.

The bus stopped at his stop, the one under the billboard sign for Alexie Life Insurance and near the place where they had taken out the old walnut tree two days before. There was a big mud hole there now. Hector spit in it, and he imagined on the walk home that his spit could sprout the tree back and he thought about the woman he'd cheated on Leda with.

They'd touched that tree together, he and the woman, as children. They'd climbed it and scraped the skin up and down their legs. His old house was down the street from where his apartment was now. Move away and move back, a little older. A paralegal now, not a scabby-kneed kid. It was as if he were on a swing set, swinging a little higher each time but always ending up in the same place. The place was different, though. Graffiti and loitering teens. Gunshots some nights, but never right outside the building. The traffic was faster now, like a little interstate, and no kids played outside here. He could've gotten a better place nearer work, but he didn't mind the noise. He only feared when Leda was walking to and from her car, so he'd walk with her, holding her hand or carrying her groceries up to his apartment. He could see the house he grew up on from the bus stop, an old box where it had just been Hector and his mom. Of course, the neighborhood was quieter then. While she had warned him to stay away from gangs, it was only in a sideways kind of way. Now, there were sirens sometimes, just sometimes, though, and he could deal with that.

Rosalie still lived here, he discovered a year after moving back. She called him up one day, had looked his number up in the phonebook, and said, "I'm outside your window. Come

play with me." And there she was. She'd gotten tall, sounded tall even over the phone. She was a teacher now, she said. She was divorced. She was doing okay. He was busy and said they'd catch up later. Leda said she was going to set the table for supper, if he was hungry. He waved to Rosalie through the window, and she smiled at him.

Leda was in Las Vegas for her sister's wedding the weekend that he and Rosalie met up. He'd had appointments, meetings and things and had to stay home. He hadn't planned on meeting Rosalie. It'd been fine just seeing her through a pane of glass, but she'd called him again on Friday during work, this time on the cell number he'd given her. He left earlier than usual to catch a drink with her. They'd had beers. Hector had always wanted to kiss a woman who could talk beer with him. Hops and malts and carbonation for an hour or so, plus her job and his. So glad to be done with school, they said. Real world, nothing like it, they said, and they hopped into a cab and had sex on the couch that Leda'd picked out. He told Leda everything when she got back in town. They sold the couch, his idea, not hers.

She'd be over at her parents' by now. Her mother would be making coffee and heating up the curling iron. They had practiced doing her hair twice a week for three weeks. Most likely, she'd be trying her wedding dress on before they left it at the church overnight. He knew Leda, the way she slipped into it and spun around in front of the mirror. It was a tiered cake of fabric,

two sizes too big before they'd had it fitted. It wasn't any less of a waterfall of lace now, but it was fit so that her pencil frame almost had curves.

Leda loved the story of the dress. She used to work at the dry cleaners and the dress had gone unclaimed for two years; two years of her staring at it. Even when they had contacted the owners, no one came for it. So when she quit, the day he proposed, she took it with her. It was an adopted child.

He'd met her there, at the dry cleaners. Right before his law school interviews he got both of his suits pressed, and when he picked them up, he asked for Leda's number. A story to tell their children about the importance of pressed clothing.

Hector's phone rang as he climbed the stairs to his apartment. It wasn't Leda, though more often than not she called just when he thought about her. He clicked his cell open. "Joey, thanks for ditching me."

Joey laughed. "How's your hangover?"

"I feel like I've been body-slammed by a whale." Hector unlocked the door to his apartment. "I'm wearing my cousin's clothes. I'm in a whole bunch of camo right now. I must be invisible."

"You need a ride to the rehearsal or are you going to have your shit together enough to catch your bus?"

"The bus is fine. See you there," Hector said.

"Don't forget to change out of that camo."

Hector turned the television in the living room on loud enough so that he could hear it from the shower. Hell, the neighbors can yell. They usually do. Yelling like a bell tolling out the hours, inside their apartments and out on the street. Hector wasn't a yeller, Leda neither, but they'd listen. The crack-whores shouting at the birds outside. Barely-licensed boys in cars going by, shouting at the crack-whores. They'd make love with the sound of the downstairs neighbors, two old men, yelling at each other about the water bill. Being in bed with Leda made him feel like he was in a bunker looking out. Yelling was better than birdsong, better than silence. It was the same with the bus. He'd always preferred the bus. Even as a child, he'd ridden it when he got an allowance. His mother always laughed. "Only people who never ride the bus love it," she always said. "They love it like tourists, kid." But he loved the shades of people, each staring at something else, and the noise of the beast below him.

In the shower, he thought about waking up. He thought he'd been in Rosalie's bed, how he'd imagined Rosalie's bed, white and clean with that scent of peonies. The two of them used to play in her family's garden as kids, picking the ants off of the peonies. Those ants ate away at the green jackets of the flowers until the head popped out, pink or white or red like a fragrant firework. When they were seven or eight, he'd dared Rosalie to eat an ant, but she wouldn't, so he dared her to eat a peony instead. She took a bite of it like an apple so that the petals fell from her lips when she laughed and said, "This is so gross." She blew the rest of the petals out of her mouth at him.

He had told Leda about the beer night right after it happened. She cried. He wished she'd screamed and thrown something at him, something heavy. But she had only cried, and they weren't even loud tears. Goddamn Leda and her long black hair and her quiet moods and her unpronounceable Greek last name.

Almost one now, and he knew he should eat but couldn't. Hector toweled himself off and wished she would call. He knew Leda was busy getting ready for the rehearsal and it made him feel guilty. He should be too busy with things too, but her family had hijacked every aspect of the wedding. Hector hadn't had a say in anything since he asked Leda to marry him. His mother hadn't put up a fight to be involved at all. Planning wasn't her specialty, hell, his very existence had been a bit of a surprise to her. A happy accident.

He sat in the armchair in the living room naked and watched ESPN. Last week, Leda'd leapt on top of him in this chair and tickled him until he was finally ticklish. The two of them toppled off together, laughing and digging their fingers into each other's sides. That was his Leda.

When Leda had had a lump scare during his first year of law school, he'd driven two and a

half hours just to hold her, reassure her, breathe with her. On her bed they lay together, one of his hands on her left breast, the other gliding up and across her stomach. The momentary realization of her fragility scared him; he said he loved her. But away from her, on the drive back at four in the morning pushing through the star-strung landscape, he didn't think. There was nothing.

One-fifteen. Everything about a wedding was pressing and inconvenient: too much or too little time. He paced in front of the window of his apartment. He thought about taking a walk outside but was afraid of running into people he knew. He called Leda's apartment instead, and the phone rang and rang.

She didn't have a machine. The ringing was comforting, though, and the waves of it washed over him. He hung up feeling better, but not knowing exactly what he was feeling shitty about in the first place.

Not the wedding. He wanted more than anything to marry Leda. He couldn't sleep without hearing her fervent whispered prayers before bed. He loved that she thought he didn't notice them. He loved her cold hands. He loved the smile that she gave strangers and how it wasn't the smile that he got. He wondered what she thought about him sometimes, thought in the secret way that he thought about her. She seemed to see through him most times, but he knew that he could keep things from her, even lied about little things sometimes just to make sure. The nights that they slept apart, he'd go

on long walks and buy little things in drug stores, kitschy things that when she asked about them, he'd make up some fantastic inheritance story. Maybe she didn't believe him but it didn't matter. He wished it felt different when he lied to her than when he told the truth. He got her same smile either way.

He saw Rosalie twice after beer night. Twice more that he didn't mention to Leda, after the couch had already been sold. The living room looked a little empty without it, but Hector didn't mind the bareness.

He hadn't meant to see Rosalie, but she was his neighbor, after all. Two insomniacs out on the same block, walking. What's unnatural about that? So what if they had been lovers, so what if she'd sucked his big toe and laughed when he said that it was the stupidest and funniest thing anyone had ever done to him. Insomnia made him crazy and hungry, and she said pancakes. Then there she was, her long legs wrapped around his waist in the bathroom of Denny's. They laughed like two potheads, swayed and almost fell together. That was the first time since the couch. The second time, late last week, he'd called her. Leda was with her parents, triple and quadruple checking the set up of the little inn where they would hold the rehearsal dinner.

"She's pretty," Rosalie said, pointing to a portrait of his girl. There were pictures of her all over one of the walls of his apartment. They were in a cascading line from corner to corner, her half-smiles, her green bathing suit. If he'd

wanted to pray, if he'd been the kind who did, he could have knelt down and faced Leda.

"Am I prettier than her?" Rosalie asked.

She wasn't. "You're different," he said. "It's like apples and oranges."

"That's a dumb cliché. Everyone has a preference." She straddled his crotch and started to bite his ear. When he didn't say anything after a minute, she sat up, propping herself up with her elbows. "I don't just do this to every guy. It's all for you, you know. For God's sake, the last thing I need is you wrecking yourself over me. Or me over you."

They were on a blanket in the middle of the floor. He'd made a fort with Leda once with that blanket before he'd fully unpacked in this new apartment and they'd made salami sandwiches to eat underneath it.

"Do you want me to stay?" Rosalie asked.

"Yes."

"Why?"

He'd tried to think of a way to tell her about the woman he'd seen on the bus, the one that he swore he knew. He had moved to sit behind her, which wasn't hard because the bus got busier and the crowds were pushing everyone together. As he was sitting near her, trying to place this woman, about to speak to her, he realized that it was just the smell of her, the same scent that Leda used, and the woman's eyes were a similar shade of grey as Leda's. All of these little things that added up to his palms beginning to sweat. He almost asked for her number, this pseudo-Leda, just to try and kiss in another woman all of these little pieces of Leda. This stranger, this strange woman on the bus, and he could almost picture her naked, centerfold-like, sprawled on the bus seats, curls of hair falling on her breasts.

But with Rosalie, it was her lips. Even lying here now, he pictured peony petals spill from them, and her laugh. "I love your lips," he'd said to her, and she'd curved them into a smile for him, a different kind of smile where she bit her lip and it curled like water under the bite. They had sex again and she left, and when she left, everything about her left, the smell and taste of her. He liked that about Rosalie.

One-forty five. He felt like he hadn't been a bachelor since the day he met Leda, like the ceremony had taken place with the passing of the receipt for his suits with her name scribbled on the back. He knew the way these things were supposed to happen, and Eve wasn't supposed to fall in love with the snake, and the snake, with Eve. He hated the forced Biblical metaphors that came into his mind when he thought about a woman that loved him enough to pray for him with him lying inches away, listening, knowing that she must know that he can hear.

If there was a God, Leda, Hector thought, I'd be killed right now to spare you. A meteor or a strike of lightning seemed fitting. Or I could miraculously devolve and tomorrow Leda'd find a slug on the floor and figure it was His will.

Ten minutes before the right bus came by to catch to the rehearsal. I could, he reasoned,

attempt to smoke 5,000 cigarettes in these ten minutes and get lung cancer and shrivel up. Maybe if I'd had at least one pack I could've gotten started.

He changed into a pair of khakis that Leda liked and a parsley-colored polo. It felt strange that Hector didn't need to bring anything with him. A comb, maybe? He could slip one in his pants pocket. He was leaving here with empty hands. Tomorrow, he'd come back with Leda in his arms. She'd begged him to carry her across the threshold. He'd done that for her already, the first night she came over and he ruined her for the rest of humanity. After law school, three years of earning her, winning her, and he'd won her on the green cotton sheets that he loved so much. When he closed his eyes, when he thought of things, most things were superimposed on her naked torso. He could hear her like an echo in other people's voices.

She knows about Rosalie, he thought. She must know. I am a terrible person. A crazy person. He shoved a comb in his back pocket and walked to the corner with the mud-hole and waited.

On this corner, there were two drunks flipping a coin on the bench, each taking a turn, going back and forth. It spun between them like a top when the taller one dropped it. There was a black woman in a sweatshirt with her son, a little boy in big pink sunglasses. He laughed at those sunglasses, the size of them on the boy's nose.

I am taking a cross-town bus to my rehearsal, he thought, and a limo from it, and he laughed. The little boy's sunglasses fell off when he bent over to pick up the penny. Hector was still laughing, tears coming out of his eyes, he felt like he was losing it. His head hurt from the laughing, being right here by the mud hole that had been his tree, his favorite tree, staring across at Rosalie's house, the absurdity of the damn comb in his pocket and how this little object could take on so much significance when tied to a wedding.

In a moment, the bus would come. He thought he could feel its treads reverberate down the street like a boy feels the big wave coming from his spot on the sand. It was moments like this, these empty spots between the entire days that they spent together that made his guts contract. It was like he lost sense of where he was without the guidepost of Leda. Did people love like this, with a guilty, endearing frustration?

The bus slowed to a stop and he watched the people board. One drunk pushed the other up the stairs. The mother grabbed her son, whose sunglasses stayed on the pavement though he pulled against her arm to reach them. His bus would leave, and he couldn't unglue his feet.

The bus pulled away with a gasp and puff, and he sat on the curb and whispered a prayer. He hadn't prayed in fifteen years. His mouth was hot. He felt that she would know, was probably praying the same words and like a canon, a round, echoing each other. Waves washing upon him, the moons of dead streetlights watching him, Hector put his head in his hands and waited for something to happen.

GOODNIGHT NOBODY

CURTIS SMITH

Magical moments in literature, take one: Gregor Samsa's horrified awakening; Colonel Aureliano's memory of ice as he stood before a firing squad; the silky billowing of Gatsby's flung shirts on the rainy afternoon he was finally reunited with Daisy.

Any book lover could run a finger along the spines of his shelved collection and feel the tug of a hundred scenes so alive they beg to be pulled out and read again.

But for me, few scenes are more profound than a two-word passage from *Goodnight Moon*. What this story of a little bunny drifting off to sleep lacks in plot, it atones for in poetry, in its induced state of mantra-driven bliss. Goodnight, clocks and goodnight, socks. Goodnight, kittens and goodnight, mittens. Goodnight, red balloon. Perfect, the mesh of the narrative's dreamy rhythms and the gradually dimming bedroom scenes. The words—few and simple—shimmer with a Zen-like grace, a fitting harmony for bedtime's wind-down fizzle.

Yet three-quarters of the way through, an impish and deceptively powerful about-face turns the narrative—and, in essence, the reader's perceived world—inside-out. The page is blank, a masterstroke of intuition and Dada-esque pranksterism. Two words grace the white field—*Goodnight, nobody*.

Goodnight, nobody. It both affirms (the acknowledging "Goodnight") and denies ("nobody"), and behold, the linguist's Mobius strip. Physicists who fret over tears in the space-time continuum should examine this self-negating, two-

word sentence, for it acts as a chain reaction's first split atom, and the unleashed force that radiates from its origin ripples out and engulfs the child's world, bestowing upon it a new dimension that will haunt the rest of his days. "Goodnight, nobody" lends weight to the weightless. It paints the invisible. In an uttered breath, ghosts are born, spirits recognized. "Goodnight, nobody" resonates as a grinning bass note smuggled into a lullaby's slumbering melody. Too young to realize it, the child has been introduced to monsters in his closet, imaginary play friends, stuffed animals that stir to life after goodnight kisses and whispers of sweet dreams.

And this netherworld of haunted non-existence echoes into adulthood, its roots burrowing deeper, twisted barbs that embed themselves in our souls and minds, filling us with an acutely individual awareness of angels and demons, of fates and forces beyond our control. "Goodnight, nobody" is a Pandora's Box of perception and awareness, a hailing of sparkling possibilities, a whisper of longing and regret and desires unfulfilled.

I read the story to my son, once, twice, again, his eyes and limbs growing heavy, a sinking into the realm of dreams he alone experiences. Goodnight, nobody, and welcome, my little man, to the unseen world, a greeting as gentle and embracing as the kiss I plant on your dozing head.

INTERVIEW: DAVID WAIN

WHAT HAVE YOU LOST THE MOST SLEEP OVER IN YOUR LIFE?

David Wain: When I was in my early 20s I felt a lot of general uneasiness in my life and my thoughts tended to spiral at night. Combined with no particular place I had to be in the morning (i.e. unemployed) I didn't get a lot of sleep.

DO YOU HAVE ANY ROUTINES OR REMEDIES FOR WHEN YOU CAN'T SLEEP?

David Wain: It hasn't been my problem in a long time, thankfully. Pretty much if I get in bed and start reading, my eyes cross within a few minutes and then I'm asleep. If I need to go to sleep at a strange hour or on a plane—then I'll take a pill.

THROUGHOUT YOUR CAREER ARE THERE ANY PARTICULARLY FOND (OR AWKWARD OR ANYTHING REALLY) MEMORIES OF SHOOTING A SCENE IN A BED?

David Wain: I remember shooting a scene for *Wainy Days* (Episode "Zandy") where it was a bed that was very much like the bed I really slept in when I was single—covered in books and newspapers and laundry; a naked lightbulb on a cord just lying there on the bed because I didn't have a regular lamp; and sheets that haven't been washed in a long, long time.

WHERE'S THE STRANGEST PLACE YOU'VE EVER SLEPT?

David Wain: I've slept just about everywhere—in every classroom I've ever been in, nearly every movie or play, watching U.S. Congress in session, in the director's chair while shooting, while driving a car, on my first date with my now wife (ALL TRUE).

YOUR DREAMS AND WHAT THEY MEAN

ANGI BECKER STEVENS

The man in Amelia's dreams was not necessarily the man *of* her dreams.

In fact, it took her a while to even notice him. He wasn't her type; he was short, on the thin side, his dirty blonde hair was just starting to thin. She tended to prefer men

men taller, darker, with a little more meat on them. This man wasn't someone she would have given a second glance, except that he was somehow familiar to her. On a dream-airplane one night, she kept stealing glances across the aisle trying to decide if he was an old schoolmate, a neighbor, a waiter she saw regularly. A few nights later, when she found herself sitting down next to him on a strange misshapen and brightly painted park bench, she realized he was simply a recurring character in her dreams.

"Hi," he said to her. "I'm Andrew."

"Amelia," she replied.

Three children ran by, all blonde and laughing, being chased by a kangaroo.

★ ★ ★

The first morning after Kate camIn the morning, she lay there in bed for a long time, rubbing her eyes, watching the sunlight advance down her wall, thinking how lately, her dreams had become awfully strange.

★ ★ ★

The first morning after Kate camBefore the man appeared, Amelia had never been one to have the meandering, fanciful dreams she often heard described. When she remembered her dreams at all, they were mundane. Scenes from her everyday life, with only minor transgressions. A kitchen she had never seen before, but understood in the dream was supposed to be her kitchen. Her car sometimes a different color. Even the occasional nightmare betrayed no subconscious sense of adventure. No imagination. A man would chase her. She would be running. Her sleeping mind never conjured monsters, intricate plots.

If a friend or co-worker gave a detailed account of a strange or hilarious dream, Amelia suspected he or she was making it up. Sure, a car shaped like a carrot, tunnels below the whole city, your dog started to speak…

What would the motive be for inventing dreams?

Amelia wasn't sure. She just couldn't believe that real people actually dreamt such things. That other minds could go places so unlike her own. That there could be such variety. Such possibility.

But the man in Amelia's dreams ushered in a new era. Her dreams became odd, silly. Colors were more vibrant. People walked goats on leashes, bottles of cream soda grew like apples on trees.

One night, she met the man at an amusement park. It was a warm, sunny day, but the two of them appeared to be the only guests there. The roller coasters ran empty. The man, Andrew, walked beside her. He stopped at one of those stands that usually sold lemonade and elephant ears and cotton candy. He bought her a balloon. Yellow, tied to a string.

"Here," he said. "This is for you."

"Thank you." She held out her hand. He tied the string around her wrist, like she was a child.

"It's strange how you keep showing up in my dreams," she said. "I don't know you from anywhere else, do I?"

"What do you mean, *your* dreams?" he asked her. They stopped walking. They stood there looking squarely at each other, her balloon quivering slightly in the breeze.

"What do you think I mean?" she asked. "I mean what I said. My dreams."

"But they aren't your dreams." He laughed. "They're mine."

"But you're a figment of my imagination!" she said.

"No I'm not! I'm a regular person, I'm back home asleep in my bed right now, flesh and blood."

"I don't believe you," she said. "Prove you're real!"

He laughed again, and she felt angry. How could he be so amused at a time like this? "How do you propose that I go about proving it?" he asked. "Prove *you're* real!"

She looked down at her feet on the ground, but they were only her dream feet, on the dream ground. She'd never been asked to defend her

existence before. Where was the evidence? She'd made no impact on the world. She felt suddenly small. Too slight to leave footprints.

"Hey," he said. "Don't look so sad. It can't be that bad, being imaginary. It'll spare you a lot of pain and suffering, if you ask me…"

"But I'm *not* imaginary!" She shouted. The tone of her voice surprised her. Shrill and desperate. Like she was fighting for her life.

"Okay, okay," he said. "I apologize. I take it back. You're as real as I am." Condescending, she thought. Like he didn't really believe her at all. She wished she could take a knife and cut into her skin. Show him how alive she was. How she bled. But it would only be her dream skin. Her dream blood. It might be blue, green, purple. Squirting from her dream veins like a Technicolor geyser. It wouldn't prove anything.

★ ★ ★

The first morning after Kate camIn her waking hours, she thought about what it meant to be real. She pondered metaphysics. Walking the streets of her town, she had the urge to throw rocks through store windows. To scream "fire!" into a crowd. To know that she could cause a reaction. To discover the weight of herself in the world.

She went into the bookstore. Embarrassed, she went to the New Age section. Quickly and without browsing, she grabbed a book called *Your Dreams and What They Mean*. When she went to pay, she laid it face down on the counter. As if it was porn.

At home, she left the book in its bag all evening. Before bed, she finally took it out. Wasn't sure where to look. She turned to the entry for "Stranger." According to the book, seeing a stranger in her dreams represented a repressed part of herself. Or a dream-helper, who was trying to offer insight.

The book didn't tell her what it meant to dream of a real man. Or to dream that she wasn't real. She imagined an entry where the book would suggest: *see a psychiatrist.*

★ ★ ★

The first morning after Kate camThat night, they were on the roof of a building somewhere, drinking wine. In the distance, fireworks. All red and purple and white.

"I've been thinking," she said. "Maybe we're both real." He wasn't looking at her, or at the exploding sky. He was folding a piece of blue paper into the shape of a bird. He threw it into the air and it flew away.

"How could we both be real?" he asked. He sounded sad. He was usually so happy. Laughing. She wasn't sure why the reality of her would have the opposite effect.

"Why can't we both be real?" She asked.

"And both dreaming?"

"Sure," she said. "Dream sharing. A dream mash-up."

He shrugged. "I never thought of that before." He kept looking off, far away. Amelia thought he liked her better when she was pretend.

★ ★ ★

The first morning after Kate cam *Your Dreams and What They Mean* told her that fireworks were a symbol of her creativity. Or, they represented her pent up and repressed feelings.

Dreams were apparently all about repression. She cursed Freud. Tried not to wonder, like a crazy woman, what Andrew thought of her.

★ ★ ★

The first morning after Kate cam "So you think this is, what, some R.E.M. dating service?" he asked her one night. They were walking along a beach, their feet bare in the sand. The sun was setting, the sky and water streaked with colors too bright for nature, though she'd seen sunsets when she was awake that looked more like paintings of sunsets instead.

"Who said anything about dating?" she asked. She thought about how he wasn't at all her type. She felt a little tingle under her skin, anyway. She must have shivered at the sensation.

"Cold?" he asked her. "Or just shuddering at the thought?"

"I'm not shuddering," she said. "But it isn't very practical, is it?" He didn't answer. She let him hold her hand. Weaving his fingers between hers. A flock of paper birds flew across the sky. The shape of a paper V. So close to the sun, she thought they might burst into paper flames.

★ ★ ★

The first morning after Kate cam They met every night, in places that were ordinary and strange. She often forgot details of the words he said. Could picture only his mouth moving. Her own face dissolving into laughter. When they walked beside each other, their feet fell into perfect synchronized rhythm.

He hummed sometimes. The tune would stay in her head for days.

★ ★ ★

The first morning after Kate cam Once, they were walking the streets in her town. A perfect summer evening. In the graffiti-covered alley on Liberty, a monkey on a leash was doing tricks. The man at the other end of the leash was dressed like a mime. White face. Black clothes. He held dozens of balloons, passing them out to any old woman who walked by.

"This is where I live," Amelia said. "More or less, I mean."

"This is where *I* live," Andrew said.

She shook her head. "I don't believe you." Of all the dreams, in all the world. It never occurred to her that such a collision would have happened with someone so close by.

"On the weekends, there's a man with a boombox in the alley," he said, "impersonating Michael Jackson."

"People say he's really a lawyer," she said. "That he just does it for fun."

"Urban legend, I think," he said. She looked down at the monkey. It did a back flip.

"But you never know," she said. "It could actually be true."

★ ★ ★

The first morning after Kate camSome nights, she couldn't wait to fall asleep. She drifted off smiling. Flutters of anticipation in her chest. Some nights, she tried to put sleep off as long as possible. Things felt turned around. Her daytime life felt trite and without consequence. In dreams, she faced reality. The heaviness of feeling.

Sometimes she thought she was falling in love with him and other times she thought she was only getting used to him, and sometimes she wondered if there was really any difference between the two.

She thought about existence. Hers. His. The world's. How once, the universe could have fit into a thimble. Maybe it still could.

She wondered how she had ever imagined that she was certain of anything.

★ ★ ★

The first morning after Kate camSometimes, the dreams they had were a strange experiment in accidental compromise. When he fell asleep thinking of fishing and she drifted off planning her shopping list, they found themselves in a rowboat navigating flooded grocery store aisles, like a walled-in, fluorescent-lit Venice.

"There are no fish here," he sulked. He was looking down into the water, his oars still.

"I'm sure there are some in the freezer section," she said.

"Har har," he said. "Would it kill you to fall asleep thinking about something a little more exciting every once in a while?"

"I didn't ask to be cosmically handcuffed to you," she said. "Now are we just going to sit here, or are you going to row me to the cereal aisle?"

★ ★ ★

The first morning after Kate camAccording to *Your Dreams and What They Mean*, dreaming she was in a rowboat was a symbol of hard work and perseverance. Also, that she was coping with things in her own way. Consider the condition of the water, it said.

Under grocery store, it said: *see market*.

To dream of being in a market represented a physical need she was lacking. Or perhaps she was feeling a lack of nurturance and fulfillment.

Dreaming of cereal indicated the beginning of a new stage in life. Or the need to restore

herself in some basic way. Alternatively, it could just be her mind thinking ahead to breakfast.

★ ★ ★

The first morning after Kate camShe tried to think of mountains, after that. Rainforests. White water rafting.

She managed only the occasional camping trip, where the land was flat. The water still.

"At least you're trying." He kissed her forehead. He handed her a bouquet of balloons. She let them go, watching them become smaller and smaller against the violet sky.

★ ★ ★

The first morning after Kate camShe looked up "Balloons" in *Your Dreams and What They Mean*. She read that they represented her declining hope in the search for love.

Ascending balloons: her desire to escape.

She closed the cover. She threw the book in the trashcan. Dumped coffee grounds on top for good measure.

★ ★ ★

The first morning after Kate camAndrew folded paper turtles and let them swim away. He folded paper snowflakes. When he threw them up into the air, real snow fell back down. It left a powder on everything. The paper dust wasn't

even cold or wet on her bare arms. They fell into it, laughing. Wanting never to get up.

★ ★ ★

The first morning after Kate camOne night, she found herself standing in front of him naked. She looked down at her body. Her breasts were a bit larger than in real life. Her stomach a bit more tight. Not much. Just a bit.

"Flattering," she said. "Reality would disappoint you." The room they were in was empty. Dim.

"I bet I'm not that far off," he said, and she smiled because he was right.

"I'm sorry for taking your clothes off," he said. "I've had a few drinks."

"I don't mind." If he had dreamed her as some kind of stick-thin model, she would have minded then.

"Where the hell are we?" he asked. "There's no furniture. I should have candles… Something…" As he spoke, there was a bed. Soft blankets. Candles on nightstands.

"Like magic," she said. When he kissed her, she was disappointed by how unreal she felt. How she lacked solidity.

"I have to warn you," he smirked. "In my dreams, I'm *damn* good in bed."

They tumbled into the blankets. Into a blurry sort of bliss. Somewhere outside of consciousness. Between reality and unreality.

She woke up feeling satisfied and sad. Touched the empty space next to her. Tried and

tried, but couldn't manage to drift back into sleep.

★ ★ ★

The first morning after Kate camThey made love in lavish hotel suites, on beaches, in the backseats of parked cars, on floors and on grass and in lakes. But aside from the sometimes-exotic locations, she was relieved that his fantasies were what she considered within the realm of normal. Things she would do even when awake.

Her life was backwards. When she was awake, she fantasized about being asleep.

In the morning, she always wanted to smash her alarm clock with a hammer. She'd never felt such hatred for an object. She pulled the blankets tight around herself. Felt loved. And alone.

★ ★ ★

The first morning after Kate camIn a hot air balloon one night, she watched the ground drift by. Slow and far away. She held onto the edge of the basket tightly. As if she could fall.

"You have the lamest flying dreams I've ever heard of," he said. She slid away from him, hurt. It could have been romantic.

"What's so lame about them?"

"They're dreams," he said. "You can fly without a vehicle if you want. You've always got airplanes. Balloons."

"Balloons are symbolic," she said. "Supposedly. I'm giving up all hope of finding love."

"Are you?" he asked.

"Yes. No. I don't know."

He took a dollar out of his pocket—the wrong color, like Monopoly money or a transient bill from Canada—and folded it into a ring. He slipped it on her finger. She sighed. She could feel it there, but just barely. If she waved her hand, the ring would flutter away, like a paper bird.

He tried some kind of joke, but neither of them was in the mood.

"I don't think we can keep doing this," he told her finally. She looked away.

"I don't think it's up to us, is it? I don't know how we can break up…"

"I'm not talking about breaking up." She looked back at him. "I think we should meet in person. Awake."

"Can we do that?" she asked.

He shrugged. "We can try."

They made their plans. A certain coffee house, at a certain time the next day.

"I'll bring a balloon," he said.

★ ★ ★

The first morning after Kate camThe next afternoon, before leaving the house, she kept looking at herself in the mirror. Checking her teeth for lipstick. Wondering what she was about to go do.

She was half convinced she was going off to discover once and for all that she'd gone mad.

But then there was the other half of her, the better half. The part she hadn't known about until the man appeared in her dreams. That half of her knew how it would be. That she would walk into the coffee house to find a certain familiar man. A certain familiar light in his eyes. He would tie a string around her wrist. A yellow balloon. She would feel light enough to float away. But she wouldn't, not really. Because that's the sort of thing that only happens in dreams.

Half a block from the coffee house, she could already see it through the window: a splash of bright yellow latex. A tiny captive sun. The yolk of an egg.

What she felt was a strange sort of calm.

What she wondered was, when they lay together in bed, all flesh and blood and bone, would they become any more real to each other than they already were?

She stopped outside the coffee house door. She pinched her arm, until her fingernails left perfect crescent moons in her skin.

When she was satisfied she was awake, she opened the door. She stepped in, aware of the air she displaced. Her presence in the room. The weight of her whole life compressed so tightly, it could become the universe.

AN UNWANTED CASKET

SUSAN L. LIN

Secrets collect underneath my bed the way dust might if I didn't clean. They settle over the floorboards like a blanket, thick enough for me to run my index finger through it, drawing a path from one point of my life to the next.

My best friend and I had matching backpacks in kindergarten. They were designed in the same style, hers with the characters of *The Wizard of Oz* on the front pocket, mine with Ariel from *The Little Mermaid*. For some reason, her backpack is the one I find when I hike up the bed skirt and look underneath. The purple PVC has a goldenrod trim and the words "Follow the yellow brick road!" written along the top opening.

Unzip the bag and the contents could swallow a room:

- *A half-used bottle of pearly blue nail polish.* No idea where that one is from. I shake the bottle like I always do to hear the tiny silver balls clink against the glass. Dried. Oh well. I toss it aside. My arm jerks a little and I throw it too far—the bottle slides across my bedspread and over the edge.

- A *nightlight with a stained glass butterfly covering the bulb.* I pick it up too quickly and cut myself on a chipped corner. This one I remember, I think, touching

a tissue to the cut. Cody Singleton's, seventh grade. I found it in his room. "It ain't mine, I swear," he kept saying. "I don't need no light to sleep at night. It's my little sister's." I didn't really give a damn whose it was. It was in his room. I said, "Your grammar sucks, you know that, right?" Now I set the butterfly down on the bed and watch the sunlight hit the glass from the outside. The colors! They fall onto my hands, dyeing geometry on my skin.

- *An assortment of writing instruments*: two ten-color pens with cerulean plastic bears on the ends, one blue pen shaped like a folded up umbrella, six blue, green, and pink push pencils, one pen with miniature dice inside a clear plastic tube, two pens shaped like red swords, three sparkly crayons, all the same shade of blue. Christ, there are so many. I spread them all out in front of me, arranging them by color, then by age. My fingers start to feel numb as I wrap them around one of the crayons, my grip slipping over the textured paper covering. I open the mouth of the bag and see what's next.

- *A blue glow-in-the-dark pen*. Mallory's, third grade. She still doesn't know.

Guilt bubbles to the surface, through the hole of a wand. I push it back out to the other side. I'll feel it again when I room with Mallory during her first year of college, but I can rationalize it away, I always do. It's not like I'll ever take anything from her again anyway.

- *A silver butterfly pendant, outlined in sapphires*. This one is wrapped in three layers of tissues and kept inside an old cookie tin. I see my blurred reflection in the lid but can't make out any features. My whole body is shaking and I don't know why. I fold the paper back over and stuff it at the bottom of the bag, everything else on top.

Minutes later, I remember the nail polish on the floor and reach over on my stomach to pick it up. My legs stretch out from under me, my feet pointed. The first time I ever see someone die, the hospital speakers will be playing Christmas carols, a glass of eggnog on the table next to me. I'll remember looking down at my feet, pointing and flexing them, making sure I'm still in control of my body.

Right now, I don't think I am: when I try to lie perfectly still, my teeth jump around in my mouth like bones trapped in an unwanted casket.

MOST OF ALL I WISH I'D SAID, IF YOU COME BACK, DON'T COME BACK TO ME

MARGARET PATTON CHAPMAN

We had only been sleeping together for a couple of months when he died of a sudden, inexplicable, deadly illness with no known treatment which killed him before I'd even heard

he'd been hospitalized. The day after he died a friend of a friend let me know, a girl I'd never met whose voice kept breaking up. I'd thought it was bad reception. She was sobbing. I didn't know what to say so I hung up and went to the bar.

"How terrible," people at the bar said.

It was terrible.

"You must be shocked."

I was shocked.

"Let me buy you a drink," said almost everyone, which is really all anyone can ever say.

The whole thing between us only started from a long stretch of desperate boredom during a particularly flat, Midwestern winter. I was looking for something, we probably both were, but neither of us had seemed all that interested in taking on someone else's insecurities and problems. And even if I did once wake up on time in the middle of the night, turn and slip my arm around him and notice how surprisingly calm and secure I felt, the unspoken rules were that this was a winter thing, that some day we'd get our summer bodies back, that one of us would go to a new bar or finally hang out with those old friends we'd been putting off, and we'd meet someone who might really make us not feel so alone.

The night after I found out, my friends Erica and Xander came over and they didn't know what to say and so we got drunk and played cards and then they left and I was alone. This sort of thing happened a few more times until it was the day of his funeral and, in the end, I didn't go. Xander said he'd take me, and Erica lent me a cute black dress, and I'd even bought pantyhose, but at the last minute I bailed. It just seemed too intimate, too awkward, because, in the end, I didn't really know him, and someone's funeral is such a big deal.

"Are you sure?" asked Erica. I was standing on my stoop, freezing in my black dress and pantyhose, smoking cigarettes and talking to her on the phone.

Of course I was sure. I'd never met his family. I'd barely met his roommate. I didn't like his dog. "I'll mourn in my own way," I told Erica. I decided this included buying a new bottle of bourbon and smoking inside the apartment.

So imagine my surprise when he came back.

To me.

It took a while to figure out what was happening. I was feeling something in my place, a sort of disoriented heaviness, but I wasn't sure it wasn't coming from me, from my own disappointments and sadnesses. I'd get up in the morning with that feeling you get when you wake up at home after returning from a long trip and you don't know where you are. I'd stare out through the frost covered windows at breakfast.

My cereal seemed particularly laden, and coffee couldn't stay warm.

Maybe two weeks after the funeral this girl I work with, Marie, came over for a beer after work. As soon as she got into the apartment I could tell that she could tell something was up, because she fingered the beaded fringe on her jacket and kept letting out tiny little moan-sighs under her breath, as if she was sensing something in some sort of hippie-ish way.

"Do you believe in ghosts?" she asked.

"I don't not believe in them," I said. It felt like a trap, because only a person who does believe would ask.

Then she said it, slowly, as if the words were creeping up for a big roller coaster drop out of her mouth. "You are being haunted."

"By who?" I asked.

"Your dead boyfriend."

"He wasn't really my boyfriend," I said.

Marie and I discussed the semantics over another beer. Though officially he and I had never been boyfriend-girlfriend, that distinction was perhaps more important before his death.

"He didn't really seem like your type," she said, then immediately looked ashamed. "No offense," she said to the apartment.

"He was good in bed," I said.

"Oh, that's too bad then," she said.

When I went to bed that night, after a few more beers and an over-the-counter sleeping pill, I felt in those last instances of consciousness

like something else was there, almost like a vibration, a hum so low you can't hear it, or soft and steady breath.

Later, when I told Xander and Erica about hippie Marie and the identification of the ghost, they both acted like they were a little bit jealous that they hadn't figured it out first.

I spent a lot of time away from the apartment after that. I went out every night, closed down the early bars, closed down the late bars too. When I was drunk enough it was easier to ignore the ghost.

About a month after he died, I decided it was time to move on. I met this guy, Sean, at a party and I invited him home. We stood smoking on the stoop for a minute before we went inside. It was snowing, and flakes covered his collar, stuck to his wispy hair. I kissed him, quickly, after he exhaled and before he could take another drag. Then we were kissing on the stoop with our cigarettes burning in our hands.

Above us, the window of my apartment rattled.

"I thought you lived alone," Sean said, breaking the kiss.

"I do," I said, not looking up, trying to play it off.

"Then what was that?" he asked.

"It's no one. Nothing," I said as the blinds raised a half an inch.

"I think there's someone there," he said, backing down the steps to get a better look.

I took his hand, "There's no one."

Upstairs something broke.

"Maybe we should call the police," Sean pulled his hand away and reached for his phone.

"No," I said, "It's just an old apartment. Come upstairs, I'll show you."

But Sean wasn't sticking around. When I got upstairs, the ghost seemed sheepish, like his dog would when it had eaten the sofa cushions after being left alone too long. In a corner of the living room, a particularly ugly hand blown glass vase lay open like a bear trap.

"I loved that vase," I said to the ghost. This was not true. I decided to clean it up in the morning.

★ ★ ★

After a week or so of invisible poltergeisting, of rattling and shaking, my dead boyfriend turned spectral. The first time I saw the gossamer whiteness of his ghost-form was in a reflection off the microwave door as I reached for a plate of nachos. I started.

"You scared me," I said, and took my nachos to the living room. His reflection in the living room window told me he followed. I turned on a nature show, glancing in the window to see if he was still with me. He seemed to grow smaller, maybe denser, but then an ant was infected by a parasite that turned it into a zombie, and I forgot to check on him, and he was gone.

He came back again the next day, fuzzy and wavering in my wonky full-length mirror. And

after that he'd be around. An image. I could place him. It was hard to see him except out of the corner of an eye, or in a moving piece of glass like the bathroom cabinet door closing or a raised bottle of beer. But it meant I couldn't even delude myself into thinking I lived alone anymore. It meant I never felt like I really had the place to myself. Instead, I was constantly reminded that he was there too now, a part of the couch not to sit on, or a light coming on, or the TV getting stuck on one channel, or the TV turning itself on and off, or the TV switching itself to baseball.

"Don't you know I hate baseball?" I said to the ghost, even though it wasn't true. I didn't mind baseball.

My friends said I should leave and find a new apartment. I couldn't imagine it would make a difference; the city is pretty easy to get around in, far easier I supposed than whatever rivers of forgetting and long shafts of light a dead man would have had to navigate to make it back to me.

"How'd that happen?" Xander asked one evening when he stopped by to pick me up, pointing to the broken vase in the corner. I hadn't even noticed it was still there.

"Guess," I said.

"Really? You know this ghost is no good," said Xander.

"Did you hear that?" I said to the ghost.

"I'm serious," said Xander.

"So am I," I said loudly, so I was sure the ghost would hear. But when we got outside

I turned back to check if the TV came on. It didn't.

"He's annoying," I said to Xander, "but he isn't that bad."

★ ★ ★

One night, about a month after the ghost showed, I was walking home from the bar, in the snow, listening to the crunch of my steps and the sound of my breath underneath my scarf, drunk enough to start to feel like these sounds were all that propelled me forward, when things started to close in. It was snowing big fluffy flakes that drifted in and out of the light. I felt, in the snow world for a moment, profoundly alone in a way that made the world seem yellowed-out into blankness. Fuck, I thought. I hope this isn't what it is like to be dead.

About a block from my house I snapped out of it when I saw a couple coming toward me, walking with dog that looked a lot like my dead boyfriend's chocolate mutt. I hated that dog, but I thought maybe I should see how he was doing, let my dead boyfriend know he was okay. The dog was on one of those extendable leashes and, when he noticed me, he strained and his walkers let him go. He came right up to me, but he didn't jump on me like my dead boyfriend's dog always would, or try to chew on my jacket. He stood in the snow, looking up at me, wagging his tail, and I pet him with my mittened hand. The dog seemed so happy and

calm, and I thought maybe the dog knew more about ghosts and how to deal with them, and so I took his face in my hands and asked him.

"Tell me what to do," I asked the dog.

The owners caught up to the dog and looked on, waiting for me to say something like, "What a sweet puppy." I held the dog's head in my hands and he was very calm, his eyes deep and still, white breath rising from his grinning mouth. He seemed on the verge of letting me know. "It's okay," I whispered in the dogs ear. "I've got him. You can tell me what to do."

"Excuse us," said the new owners as they tightened the leash and pulled the dog away before he could tell me anything.

When I arrived home, a feeling of expectancy hung about the apartment, as if he was hungry for news. As if he knew.

"I'm tired," I told the ghost. I wanted to tell him about the dog. I wanted to tell him about everything, but then I thought if he had wanted to see the dog he should have haunted those people.

★ ★ ★

Sometime in March I started seeing this sort of metal guy named Ryan. We met at a new bar that opened up in my neighborhood, and he was cute enough and funny enough that I was into him for a while. When we were lying in bed one cold, sunny Sunday afternoon, Ryan said, "I'd like to meet your ghost."

"He's not that important," I told Ryan. "And he won't like you."

"I think I would like him," Ryan leaned to kiss me.

"I don't know," I said and turned from his kiss. I didn't want Ryan getting involved in this. There was something in the way he looked when we talked about the ghost, sort of predatory, needy. Like he forgot that the ghost, as he said, was mine.

Ryan ran one of his painted fingernails along the back of my hand. "I know, I'm sorry," he said. "He must have really loved you."

"We were not in love. We weren't even really in like."

"But he came back to you. Maybe he was in love. Maybe you broke his heart. We could get a Ouija board, find out," Ryan said like he was announcing the solution to a grisly crime. It was bright, almost spring-like outside, and I was getting uncomfortable in bed.

"I have to go," I said. "I'll call you later."

And that was the end of Ryan.

★ ★ ★

I laughed when I told Erica about Ryan and the Ouija board, and she laughed too, and, as a joke, a few nights later she and Xander came over with one and a couple of bottles of wine. We sat in the middle of the living room floor, closed our eyes and let our fingers rest ever-so-gently on the teardrop-shaped plastic pointer. Nothing

happened. We tried again. We concentrated. Erica called out:

"We know you are here, why are you ignoring us?"

"Maybe he doesn't know how to use this thing," Xander said.

"He's not stupid," I said. "He could do it if he really wanted."

But the ghost continued to ignore us. Eventually the wine ran out and the two of them went home.

They left the board with me.

I was cleaning up the wine glasses and putting on my pajamas and getting ready for bed when I just knelt down at the front of it, not even touching the plastic pointer and asked, *Why?*

"Why?" I said out loud. "Why?"

The air pressure dropped, as if the room let out a long sigh. And the pointer moved. It scuttled about like a drunken mouse, weaving to spell:

I D O N T K N O W

I put my hand down to stop it moving.

"You don't know?" I was incredulous. Actually, I was mad. "You don't know? Didn't you have any place better to go?"

The pointer burrowed out from underneath my hand and wriggled to NO. A pain hit me somewhere between my eyes and my nose that I couldn't quite place. He didn't come back to me. He just came back. My eyes stung.

"But how long are you going to be here?" I asked.

Again he spelled out:

I D O N T K N O W

"Really?"

The pointer wavered, not knowing how to answer that.

"Am I supposed to be doing something for you? Helping you?" I asked.

Again:

I D O N T K N O W

"I don't want to talk anymore," I told him, and I began to get up.

The little pointer scurried over and nudged my knee. It wriggled. It flipped on its back.

"Is there something you want to say?"

Upside down, it slid over to YES.

"Go ahead." I said. "Shoot."

The mouse ran back over to me and nudged my knee again.

"Do I have to ask something?"

The mouse shot to YES again.

"Who made up these rules?" I asked with out thinking, and the mouse started spelling out "I don't know" but I stopped him.

"This is pointless," I said. "All I want to know is why you are here, and you won't tell me that."

We both stayed still, me and the pointer mouse. The whole apartment was still. I looked

at the thing, sitting there, useless and I felt bad. He obviously wanted to say something. I thought for a moment and finally asked the easiest question.

"What is it like?"

The pointer didn't move for a few seconds, and then slowly, hesitantly it spelled out:

L   O   N   E   L   Y

E   M   P   T   Y

S   T   R   A   N   G   E

He stopped spelling. I sat back on my heels. The air seemed thicker and gravity stronger but maybe it was just I couldn't do anything. I couldn't do anything to make it less heavy.

"Shit," I said. "Shit. I'm sorry. Shit."

Then, for the first time since he came back, I felt him physically, as if a hand was resting gently on my shoulder, cool and almost weightless. In the window across from me he shimmered vaguely. My ankles hurt from kneeling and the air pressure in the house was dropping again. My ears popped and I felt dizzy and all the time I could feel him, just making contact, until I realized I could lean into him a little, that he was sturdier than I thought, so I did.

We stayed there a while, me leaning into nothing, him holding me up, and it seemed like he was still trying to tell me something, like maybe he was trying to say he was sorry too, for putting me through all this. Sorry that we were stuck here together, sorry that he didn't know what to do any more than I did, sorry because if things had been different, maybe, but here we were now, the empty and lonely and strange, both of us not really knowing anything, and that was all he could say about it silently, with his ghostly touch.

FATHER FIGURINE

J. ADAMS OAKS

Lilah never slept at home. Her frameless mattress, unicorn sheets and Lulu Teddy were moved into Dolores' apartment after Lilah's father walked out. Lilah and her mother lived across the hall from Dolores, the neighborhood spinster, who'd grown old without realizing life was

passing. Working as a seamstress for one of the many Collins Cleaners in town, fixing tears, patching knees, replacing buttons, she'd spent years at a table behind the rows of dry-cleaned clothes covered in plastic at the shop down the street next to Bud's Bar and had gone home each night to eat a cold sandwich and drink a cup of tea before bed. Forced to retire several years earlier (how many, she couldn't remember), Dolores continued sewing at home for her faithful customers.

Though Dolores was just her mother's friend, Lilah called her Tia—Aunt in Spanish. Lilah explained the title to her school friends when they came over to play, though the visits were seldom. So Lilah slept in one corner of Tia's knitting room, in the company of wicker baskets overflowing with fuzzy yarn and bolts of kaleidoscopic cloth while her mother worked night shifts at Bud's.

Lilah hooked her doll-like feet over the bottom edge of the mattress and covered her head with the brown and green afghan that Tia had knitted for her. She hid, not from the amber light seeping through the door left open a crack, but from the thin solitary statue on Tia's gray stone mantelpiece that stared through the crack in the knitting room door. If Tia shut

the door, Lilah became terrified of the dark. If Tia left the door open, that little man with the black hat glared at her. His face, shadowed by the brim of his hat, and spindly black body gave her nightmares about the alley behind their building, nightmares that ended with wide-awake screams.

Lilah pretended she was a chipmunk, cozy in her burrow, so the dark was okay. If a chipmunk liked the dark and she was a chipmunk, then she could like the dark under the covers. If she needed light she only had to lift her head from under the afghan. But a pigeon fluttered its wings in the cold outside and the noise made Lilah shiver.

"Tia?" Lilah's timid voice became trapped in the bed sheet. Razor-backed dogs scraped against the window pane. Or was it robbers with sharp knives? No, Lilah decided, it was the piranha fish with legs. The pigeon cooed softly and ruffled its gray feathers. The cooing, like hunting calls of the green-scaled fish, jolted Lilah from under the warm covers to the doorknob without touching the floor and into the brightly lit living room where Tia sat sipping a cup of chamomile. The black-hatted figure, master of the robbers and piranhas, loomed on the mantel above the woman drinking steaming tea.

"Tia, Tia." Lilah latched her tiny, pale arms around the woman's mottled neck. A drop of yellow tea spilled on Tia's house dress and bled into the material. "Tia, the thing is there… The

thing. Making hoo-hoo noises. Teeth and the window. Breaking the—"

"Calm, sweetie," Tia said, shaking with the girl's sobs buried in her sloping shoulder. "Shush… shush… Calm now. Tell me what's the matter."

She carefully placed the blue tea cup on the end table against the lamp's edge and lifted Lilah's damp face to hers. Tia inhaled mild no-tears shampoo and minty toothpaste. The little girl's blurred eyes caught a glimpse of the hovering figurine, and she buried her face again.

"Come on now, Lilah."

"That man, he makes the fish come…and their big teeth to eat me." Her pudgy finger wavered toward the mantelpiece.

"Oh, honey, that figurine isn't doing anything. Come now. Listen to me. He can't hurt you."

"But he takes me to the alley. He calls the animals into my room."

"Don't be foolish." Tia unwrapped the arms from her neck, as if removing a scarf, and stood up. To Tia, the girl's fear was ridiculous. When she was much younger, Tia bought the figurine for herself. One Christmas, she'd spotted it in the jeweler's window, entered the store and paid cash. It reminded her of what her boss must have looked like, the rich man with twenty-five shops who never once visited the one where she'd worked her entire life. But she liked to imagine that if he had stopped in, Mr. Collins would have honored her devotion by taking her

away from the cleaners for the most elegant night of her life. She'd even made a long gown, just in case her daydream came true. It had taken almost a year to save up for the light blue satin and to design the pattern just so. Each stitch had been carefully pondered, each ruffle measured and arranged. Once finished, the gown flowed off of her then young body like a waterfall, splashing off her shoulder, over her hips to her pale feet. What Tia never knew, as she made the dress and waited for his arrival, was that the heavy-set Mr. Collins had died of a heartattack in his spacious commissioned bathtub years earlier and a conglomerate had purchased his small string of stores to merge it with their national chain, leaving the original name for the sake of product recognition.

Tia led the child to the fireplace. She took the figurine gently between her fingers and brought it down to Lilah's line of vision. The hat brim's shadow raised to a smiling face the size of a walnut. The figurine's sinister appearance disappeared with lamp light illuminating its every glossy feature: its tuxedo, top hat, cane, grinning emerald-eyed face, and spindly legs that had been frozen mid-saunter.

"This is Mr. Collins, the rich man. He's going to the opera."

"No, Tia," Lilah said, suddenly smiling, "That's my daddy."

"Your father?"

Lilah reached forward slowly to touch the figurine's glass hat. It *was* her father. She'd never seen the figurine close up before, but the green eyes were *his*. The black and white suit he wore to call cabs in front of the hotel was *his*.

Just before he left for good, her father came to tuck her in. She looked into his eyes as he sat on the edge of her bed. He leaned over and hugged her tightly. Lilah felt the plasticy black material of his work jacket against her bare arms. She smelled the spicy alcohol he'd patted on his freshly shaven face. She squeezed harder too, not understanding why.

"Come on, Peter, you're already late for work," Lilah's mother muttered dryly from the hallway, buttoning her winter coat.

"Do you mind?"

"Peter—" Lilah's mother blurted his name like when she said "no" to ice cream before dinner.

"Shut up," Peter barked at his wife who stood too far away to slap, "and let me talk to my daughter."

Lilah had squeezed him tighter, but he still left. That was how she started sleeping in Tia's knitting room, "So mommy can work nights at the bar and earn more money, sweetie."

"Those are daddy's eyes." Lilah grabbed the figurine from Tia. She held it close to her nose. The icy glass warmed in her grasp.

"See, Mr. Collins won't hurt you," Tia said, "He's taking you out on the town. You are going to a fancy restaurant and to a show, maybe even to the opera. And you are wearing a beautiful dress I'll make you. I'll make it with that purple cloth you like."

Tia walked the girl back to bed, letting her carry the figurine, and continued talking about the man who takes her arm and guides her into a shimmering concert hall. But Lilah didn't imagine Mr. Collins. She imagined her father taking her downtown in a taxi, her dress, the color of grape juice, swirling across the seat onto his lap.

"...and Mr. Collins brings you pretty flowers. Big yellow carnations, maybe..." Tia continued telling the story in whispers as she ran her fingers gently over Lilah's hair that spread across the pillow. The words, as warm and smooth as the flannel sheets, calmed Lilah into sleep under the afghan.

Her father in his felt top hat. Lilah in the grape juice dress which spun around her legs like a merry-go-round. But they were not in a taxi or a concert hall. The two stood in the alley behind the apartment building in the bleak glow of a street light. Her father knelt and placed his hands on her thin, shivering shoulders. He held her tightly, the purple material crinkling with his grip, whispering, "I'm back now."

Animal noises rose from the murky corners. He would protect her from the piranhas that scrambled over the fireescape, their scales rasping across the brick walls. A tomcat's yowl buzzed like flies in her ears. Lilah dug her fingers into the back of her father's jacket and looked up, but his green eyes were gone. The brim of his hat shaded them from the streetlight. The piranhas skittered toward her, their black eyes shining, and began to chomp at her crinoline hem. She squeezed tighter, but he thinned in her hold, shrinking, hardening, cooling. The piranhas' teeth devoured clumps of her dress and drew closer to her skin.

Lilah woke to a slice of light from the door. She was alone in the knitting room again except for Mr. Collins looking down at her from the bed stand. Lilah picked up the figurine and cradled him between her forearms. She cried quietly, looking into Mr. Collins' green eyes, hoping he would take her to the opera since her father was made of glass.

PERCHANCE TO DREAM

THE RESIDENTS

It's only been two weeks since Howard died, so I guess I should be destroyed, a miserable wretch, shattered and scattered like the shards of a discarded whiskey bottle after it hits the pavement. But I'm not. I'm not, you see, because nothing could be worse than watching him

die. Nothing could be worse than watching a life you love slowly being sucked away like a spider draining the brain from a fly.

No. Nothing could be worse, but something could be better. Like the night he came back. Maybe it was only in a dream. Maybe it was only in every dream I've had every night since he died, but so what? Who needs reality filled with grief when love lives in your dreams? In the past, they always quickly faded, but, since Howard died, my dreams are like permanent movies living in my mind. Every second of every dream is mine, whenever I want it.

The first night was like a lamp being lit in the blindness of a black and empty room. The flame of the lamp grew brighter and brighter until the room disappeared, replaced by his face, shining like the center of the sun. Arms grew out of each cheek, opening wide in an obvious invitation to the space between his large and blood red lips. I freely fell into the opening and, once inside, easily embraced his heart. It was stuck to the top of his torso, where the nape of his neck might have been, then it licked me with love and with laughter and made my mind twinkle and grin. The dream flowed on in its

own loose and liquid way, filling my mind with a warmly glowing wetness that always equaled the essence of Howard.

But then I woke up. And the world of the waking wasn't nearly so nice. It was black. Blacker than hatred and blacker than spite and blacker than the eyes of a shark, just before it rips your arm off. Howard's parents were arriving at noon. It wasn't bad enough that I had to relive his decline and death with each of our friends. I had to do it again with his parents. His mother had never liked me, and somehow I knew she would make me feel even more guilty and responsible than I already did. It was Howard's idea to go with me, and he took the same precautions I did, but he never was very strong, except in his soul. The visit with his parents was even more miserable than I had anticipated. With memories of the previous night's encounter still pleasantly lingering in my mind, I went back to bed as soon as they left, even though it was only four in the afternoon.

The sense of satisfaction was almost immediate. Howard was hugging me from the moment my head sunk into the softness of my succulent cloud-like pillow. Instead of assorted parts, he was a whole person this time. A whole person who was also a hole, pulling me in like a lover who hasn't tasted the sweet release in a long, long time. My body became rigid and erect like a diver slipping into the sea, and I felt myself enter his soul. In and out I went, tasting

the delicious flavor of tension and release, tension and release, until we both exploded, like overripe raisins in the sun. I lay in his arms for a few sweet forevers, until the sound of screaming opened my empty ears.

Rachel, my best friend, was waking me up to go to Howard's funeral. I had slept for eighteen hours. The heaviness of grief saturating that funeral service was more than I could bear. But I had to bear it. It didn't matter how many times I broke down or how many condolences left the lips of my family and friends. It never got any better. But somehow it managed to get worse.

Just as the service was ending, I tripped at the edge of the pile of dirt waiting to fill Howard's hole. As I tripped, I bumped into his mother, causing both of us to fall into the open grave, and giving her the only excuse she needed to release an explosion of venom and rage. As my friends and family looked on, my dead husband's mother hit me fourteen times with her purse before I fainted into the waiting arms of my beloved.

My life continued on like that for the next two weeks, as I slept a little longer and dreamed a little more each day. I made it twenty-three and a half hours yesterday, and now, with Howard's support, I think I'm ready. The doctors say it's medically impossible for a healthy person to sleep twenty-four hours a day, but Howard and I don't think so.

And that's all that really matters.

JUGS

PAMELA BALLUCK

Fade in to my life, flashing back: I'm in my eleventh year, which means I'm ten (because when you turn a number, you're not just beginning to be that age, you've completed it), and I'm still in Montana on Gramma and Grampa McGlynn's Peaceful Bay Quarter Horse ranch, where I

was born and my mother was born. I don't want to draw attention by enlisting Gramma, and my big sister Aggie is flat-chested, so I go straight past needing a training bra to stealing a 34C from Mom's dresser drawer, unwilling to risk walking through the embarrassment of her saying I'm "sexy" in store aisles or sobbing in the dressing room, "Rose, you're becoming a woman," like she did in our bathroom when Aggie started her period. If Mom had lived long enough to see me turn twelve, let alone top-off at a 37D, I wonder if I would have continued to go to such lengths, or would I have eventually let her take me bra shopping?

Flash forward a couple years, 1973, at the Pacific Palisades apartment towers that Dad, Aggie, and I first moved to after Mom died and Gramma and Grampa McGlynn left Montana for Florida. L.A. is Dad's hometown. This is where Gramma and Grampa Singer raised him and where he met Mom, where Aggie was born.

I'm tanning on a lounge by the pool, facing the ocean, in my first custom-made bikini (my top and bottom sizes no longer come in sets), and somebody's shadow falls over me. It's Dad, who does an utterly-disgusted W.C. Fields—arms, elbows, and all—then turns and stalks away. He won't come back. I can't figure it, so upstairs I noodge him until he tells

me that from his home-office window, he spotted a knock-out broad he'd never seen before, and when he went down to meet her, she was me.

Cut to: Eighteen. I re-learn roller skating and pass my boyfriend Efrem's lessons in the smooth and ramped security garage of his Santa Monica apartment. We agree I'm ready to graduate to the Venice Boardwalk. Soon we're at Pico and Lincoln, returning the rentals, and Efrem is buying me a pair of white-boot Chicago's—white toe-brakes, red wheels and laces. Sometimes I skate with Efrem in Santa Monica, but I meet Aggie at the Boardwalk every Sunday, sun or fog, where we roll in shorts and legwarmers, T-shirts and loud sweatshirts, knee pads and wrist guards, onto café patios for brunch, bricks under wheels gritty with sand, before skating north on the Speedway, then Ocean Front bike path to the Santa Monica Pier and back. And every time we skate by this one pavilion, this same bum in the shadows off the Speedway—hat brim angled down over his eyes, bottle-shaped brown paper bag on his lap—in a flat, resonant baritone says, "Jugs."

Here's what I'm getting at: Dr. Berger, out of the clear blue, asks me to consider having a "breast reduction." Have I heard of this before? No.

He makes me an appointment to see a plastic surgeon in his building, Dr. Zeitman, who examines me and tells me about the procedure, then shows me his catalogue of photographs, before-and-afters. He doesn't pressure. How unnerving. Scars shaped like anchors.

★ ★ ★

Dr. Berger—who's kind of like an uncle (he went to U.C.L.A. with Mom and Dad)—has been trying to get me to see some "realities" in relation to my breasts. "In order to do the pencil test on *you*, we'd have to use the whole *box*," (ha ha). He tells me that, at eighteen, I shouldn't jog, shouldn't play tennis, shouldn't ride horses, "or you'll give yourself a black eye," (very funny). Swimming's okay. Roller skating and cycling are semi-okay with a Jogbra. "If you don't have this surgery done, you'll be tucking 'em in your belt by the time you're thirty," (thanks, Uncle Bob).

★ ★ ★

My brain's still trying to wrap itself around the idea of the possibility of this (plus, Efrem doesn't want it and won't say—plus, I think I'm finally beginning to mean something at the production office), and now I'm supposed to make up my mind already because Dad's Writers Guild insurance won't cover me once I'm finished being eighteen (which really means they'll cover me through my nineteenth year).

So, if I do it, I'll explain this at work *how*? I'd have to talk about my boobs at the office?

Doctors Berger and Zeitman and my gynecologist, Dr. David, don't classify the reduction as cosmetic surgery. It will involve cosmetic surgery—lots—they're recommending it, though, as preventative. Cancer runs not only on Mom's

side, but on Dad's, too. If I'm back down to a B- or a C-cup, Doctors Berger and Zeitman and David predict, lumps could be more easily detected. Right now, breast exams consist of wading around in so much fibrous tissue fingertips disappear at first knuckles. Mammograms hurt—I don't care what anyone says—each pendulum viced between cold, hard plates.

Aggie, who's barely a B-cup, says, "You do this, tell them to save some for me, okay?"

What, in a jar?

Efrem listens and winces. He's as mature about this as he can be, considering it's the future of my breasts we're talking about. I don't think he's named them or anything, but I sense he wants to stomp his feet and pout.

Excuse me for being intrigued. I can make them smaller? Who knew? I'm thinking, my boobs may be a turn-on, a comfort, and beauties—somehow—to Efrem, but he doesn't have to carry them around with him. I have stretch marks beginning on my shoulders. It's a nightmare buying off-the-rack because I'm so tall and skinny. Almost everything's got to be too tight or too loose somewhere, or too old-ladyish. I'm thinking, Mom died of breast cancer. I'm thinking, this is preventative.

★ ★ ★

When I go to bed now I notice pretty consciously that when I lie on my side, say my left side, my left boob gets cradled in, overflows, the crook of my left elbow and bicep, separating boob from mattress, while my right arm nestles vertically up the center of my chest, hand below chin, the arm's inside (upside) cradling the right boob, separating it from flubbing over and sticking to the left.

Whenever I sleep next to Efrem, I'm ready to shield them from being rolled on, pinched together, pinned to the mattress or to him.

I realize I've been moving in a constant, unconscious dance of self-protection.

★ ★ ★

Giving blood at Cedars-Sinai, scheduled twice, for myself. If I need a transfusion (*infusion?*) during surgery, I get my own.

I made up my mind in time to safely bank my own blood, replenish it, recover, and have the operation before my nineteenth birthday (the nineteenth anniversary of my birthday). I know, it's fast. But this kind of surgery isn't cheap. It's major. It's now-or-never, while I can still benefit from Dad's Writer's Guild insurance, while I'm still under his roof.

I'll walk into my twenties, into the '80s, a Renaissance Woman. But, will scars be faded by the time '80 is out, before I hit twenty-one? Scars I saw in photos were still dark, pink at best. This surgery is still so innovative, still so new, the after-photos are pretty new too. Scars like anchors.

★ ★ ★

I'm warning you, this isn't pretty.

Dr. Zeitman tells me he's literally going to be removing my nipples and areolas and setting them aside, nerves and lifelines intact, so he can slice down the front and center of each breast and, below each, make a horseshoe-like incision from one side to the other, where eventually bra underwires will ride. Extracted tissue will be discarded, unless my sister wants to make arrangements on her own (leave me out of it), and what's left, once inspected, will be pushed higher and reshaped into Cs. My nipples won't be *put back*, per se, but positioned where they ought to be on the new breasts, hopefully still in working order.

Doctors Zeitman and Berger warn me the worst that could happen is nip-numbness. Though, I might regain all sensitivity, and then some.

They say I might one day even be able to breast feed.

★ ★ ★

Aggie straightens and re-cascades the coffee table magazines in Dr. Zeitman's Cedars-Sinai waiting room. Dad glares at the No-Smoking signs. He can't sit anywhere in this room and claim not to see one.

In an exam room, Dr. Zeitman marks up my boobs with black ink and blue.

In my Cedars hospital room, Dr. Zeitman's team goes over the drawn map of my surgery, standing around my bed, where I sit, topless, and

pointing pens at me—at my enormous bottom-heavy, stretch-marked, lop-sided pair of tits—adding little touches to Dr. Frankenzeitman's diagrams. And I wonder: If these guys reducing me to C-cups had seen me—encountered these boobs—in their outside worlds, say in their bedrooms, would they, *do* they, find them fine or desirable right now? As guys—not as doctors—are they feeling something like Efrem is?

Scars like anchors.

★ ★ ★

I think I was in surgery more than five hours. I can't remember—did somebody say *eight hours* between the time the anesthesiologist asked me to begin counting backwards from one hundred and I rolled my eyes at him but couldn't get much past ninety-nine and the time that I woke up in post-op to my nurse Wingate sans bow-tie, in a gown with the same print as mine? I gave him a hard time about stealing my thunder, or at least my ability to make an individual fashion statement on such an important day.

I feel wicked—I love everyone—like a benevolent, mischievous drunk being wheeled away from the bar.

★ ★ ★

My nineteenth birthday, day after surgery, and Wingate has stolen for me—"borrowed," he says, over a red-and-blue herringbone

bow-tie—a little fridge from "the Liz Taylor memorial suite" upstairs. Wingate says, "She has nothing scheduled."

People bring champagne and wine and *three* cakes: one from Dad, one from big sister Aggie ("Don't they talk?" Gramma Singer wants to know); and one from my Doppelgänger, Margot, whose dad is also in TV, whose mom also died of breast cancer in Montana, but whose own big boobs are so far hassle free and still buoy up like they're floating on water; her family's place was on Placid Bay, mirroring our ranch, around a point, on Peaceful Bay. Margot's adoptive big sister April is one of my sister Aggie's oldest friends. The Doppelgänger list goes on.

Dr. Zeitman hears the pop of a champagne cork and almost faints dead away after he walks in on me in bed opening a bottle of Cab—I should not be using my cork-pulling muscles. I offer to pour him a glass.

I think Efrem's relieved I'm feeling no pain and have such round-the-clock attention, so he could duck out, go back to the recording studio, far from the reality of what's under my gown, under these bandages, with a clean conscience. *Tubes* are coming out of me—on both sides—drainage is dripping.

It's a done deal.

★ ★ ★

I'm recuperating at home—rather than camping at Efrem's while he needs to be in the studio; rather than shifting the balance at my sister and Teige's by asking her to stay home with me, when Teige wants Aggs downtown at the factory or in the showroom—but I spend little time, except overnight, in my own bedroom. Dad's master bedroom is presentable and centrally located. Afternoons through primetime, I lie around popping pills, watching TV, French doors open to the patio, hall door open to the pool room. Dad's current project, the jazz movie, which he'll co-produce, is still in development, and he's been working Peaceful Bay Productions from home—so there's always someone around to look in on me. There's always something happening, someone coming and going. Visitors can play pool, swim, do a barbeque—become occupied with something, someone, other than me—and I don't feel so bored or so boring. I'm sure I can hear the ocean from Dad's bed, but I'm told that's impossible—it's the cars down on Sunset.

Work has stopped calling me much anymore, asking how to crack my Rolodex codes— asking, "Where's the grip-truck rental file?"—asking, "Where are the extra storyboard easels"—asking, "Where's ground gourmet?"—asking, "Where's the typewriter ribbon?" They're in chaos—shooting one commercial and casting the next—and I'm falling asleep on the phone.

But the drugs don't numb, can't erase, the new reality under this dressing I've been changing myself. It's hard to imagine I'll ever look natural or show my naked body to anyone past those who

did this to me (or *for* me—yet to be determined). I think of Mom, and how she must have felt when Dad looked at her; and how he must have felt, looking at her; half of her a scar.

I find the uglier I get in my own eyes—the Frankenzeitman stitches, and the bruises turning not only blue-purple, but *green* and yellow—the more I'm reminded, after what I've been through—which looks like a fucking car wreck so it's okay if I stand in front of the full-length and cry—I obviously have a lot of healing to do before I'll begin to recognize (hopefully), when I look in the mirror, any resemblance to a woman's real body.

★ ★ ★

My follow-up visits to Dr. Zeitman are on a schedule like this: twice, then once, then twice a week, coinciding with each new event and stage and official transition of my planned recovery. Soon, these visits will taper off, and I'll be licensed to operate the new boobs on my own for a lifetime. Meanwhile, Dr. Zeitman eagerly inspects me like I'm an important experiment. I watch his face, to see if I'm looking all right. Believe me, only he can tell.

I'm wearing, doctor's orders, soft, cotton Warner bras that hook in front. And now Dr. Zeitman measures me for a Pressure Bra—a massive, prescription, harness-like thing that will apply the right pressures to incisions, scars,

once the dressings are off—to promote better healing—not very sexy.

I'm not allowed to operate a vehicle for three weeks post surgery. I can't get to Efrem's place on my own, so he comes to me, plays laserdisc movies from his own collection on Dad's identical first-one-on-the-block machine (they shopped together). Ef's been picking me up in his old Bug, Lady—perfect, no shoulder belts—taking me to Westwood, to movies we've already seen—Louis Malle's *Pretty Baby* (that little Brooke Shields), Gary Busey as *Buddy Holly*, Warren Beatty's *Heaven Can Wait*—to check out again the scores of his competition. Last Friday after the movie he took me to his apartment for the weekend.

He's squeamish about sleeping with me, body-to-body close, but he wants me there with him.

He doesn't worry out loud about our age difference. I haven't heard "When you're twenty-one I'll be thirty-one" in forever.

He doesn't want to see me beyond the bras, but I find him staring, getting used to the new look, the new shape of me.

I don't think he'll be too squeamish too much longer.

I feel like I'm winning something over on my former boobs—my original equipment. What does that mean exactly?

★ ★ ★

Dr. Zeitman removed the visible stitches yesterday. Some sutures are left inside that will disintegrate, dissolve on their own, in time. Now I wear light tape to encourage stitchless seams growing together. My bruises have faded, and I can really see: My boobs are now covered with the same skin in the same place that used to be above the level of my nipples. Before surgery, I had a bandeau tanline level across my chest, above nipples (of course). Now the same tanline is *below* horse shoes, is a narrow band of pale skin *below* my breasts. My boobs, around areolas and nipples, are completely suntanned.

★ ★ ★

Here's how I got the black eye: I'm allowed to full-on shower again—hot water pelting me all over—and at first I'm nervous, but it's great. Standing there, like normal, soaping myself everywhere, makes me feel like one skin, one fluid body again, and showering quickly goes back to routine. Part of the routine is that, in my corner of the house, the hot water goes fast. I guess I wasn't aware of how, before, to economize, I'd rinse under each breast and corresponding armpit at the same time. Imagine a flamenco dancer. First I'd raise my right arm above my head, to offer that armpit to the water, simultaneously swinging my left hand over to lift my right boob and allow the spray access to its underside. Repeat the same motions to my left. The dance began unconsciously. Where the back of my hand went to lift up my boob, there was air.

★ ★ ★

My sister and Teige are helping me clothe my new size—my new shape—in the latest, on the cheap, straight off factory and showroom floors. Aggs has more *ins* Downtown, in the Garment District, at the Mart, now that Teige is partnered with his friend Mick in their own unisex jeans company, designing and manufacturing, instead of his repping someone else's line. I had no idea how fun it is to wear clothes! I can even dress sexy now and still look "innocent"—in tops that are gauzy, or knit—diaphanous to some extent—over nude bras or camisoles, or I can wear loud and tight—and *still* not draw the kind of attention I did when I was practically trying to hide in my clothes.

I notice—after my sister and Teige helpfully bring it to my attention—I must have been subconsciously letting my butt go in an attempt to balance myself out. But I don't need this ballast anymore. Ef says he'll get me started jogging around the Santa Monica high school track a few blocks away from his place, soon as I'm permitted. He says to call it "SaMo."

Maybe I'll even quit smoking.

★ ★ ★

Dad is hosting the "annual" Emmy-watching party he throws when he's not nominated or serving on the board of governors. The TV is on in the living room, and so are the ones in the kitchen, dining, and pool rooms.

Some of us are watching from atop and around Dad's landing pad of a bed. His agent Evelyn says, "*Ol' Red Hair is Back* is a terrible title!"

Aggie says, "Her hair's really red?"

Teige nods. "I've seen her pubic hair."

My Doppelgänger, flaunting her cleavage, asks Teige, "When have you *ever* seen Bette Midler's pubic hair?"

Teige tells Margot, "I *have*. In the showroom once."

"And this from a man," Aggie says, "who confuses Shirley Jones with Florence Henderson. God-knows whose pubic hair you're actually remembering."

"Bette Midler came into the showroom," Teige says, "and Florence Henderson didn't. She didn't close the changing-room door. It was a red triangle."

Ef says, "How can you mix up Mrs. Partridge with Mrs. Brady?"

"He gets Ed Asner and Carroll O'Connor confused too," Aggie says.

Lou Grant and *All in the Family* are walking away with it.

Except for my laughter and the blaring TV, the room goes silent. All eyes are on *me*. "What?"

Aggie winces. "You're on your belly."

I have a pillow under me. But now I'm aware of the pressure, the unnatural pull. It doesn't hurt. It's not uncomfortable, until I think about it. The idea of lying chest-down without a pillow does make me cringe, though, like Aggs.

She begs, "Sit *up*. Turn *over*."

My now medium-size boobs feel like they're part of me, but not as if they've grown from me: as if they've grown attached.

★ ★ ★

Efrem and I finally have sex, make love, fuck—the first time since surgery. I keep my bra on, for my protection and for his. "Training bra" finally makes sense to me, because Ef and I are re-learning things about ourselves and each other and about us two together, and no matter how hokey this sounds, it seems we're both literally and figuratively in training to finally bare ourselves. Plus, my nipples aren't numb—they're more sensitive than ever. For now, it's best to keep covered.

Ef wouldn't do it unless we were in the exact center of the bed and I was on top, and oh God, it's a whole other thing without those saggy, giant boobs swinging around between us.

It seems like I'm on one side of windows after curtains, old heavy drapes, have been taken down—and people on the other side can see in, see me, clearly now. And I can see them seeing me.

★ ★ ★

More amazing than the ease and rewards of buying off-the-rack: This eye-contact-thing. My boss says to me, "You're too pretty to wear so much makeup"—like he's never seen my face before. Like a film's been stripped down between us.

I feel peeled.

I can't make sense without clichés.

I feel freed.

I'm no longer using the tape, and—when I'm not home wearing the Pressure Bra—I can wear soft, form-fitting bras with no-guilt, no-fear-tight tops, like a regular person. Even tubetops (a revelation).

Our assistant director Walt watches me cross the set toward him, looks me square in the eyes, and says when I reach him, "Great tits! Congratulations!"

This observation *before* would have not been so open, wouldn't have seemed so friendly, would have been a thing I dreaded, a curse and a spell I had nothing to do with casting. *Before*, Walt would have blushed ten shades if I'd caught him even glancing at my "rack," my "melons," my "tah-tahs." But now I have tits and eye contact, which I didn't realize I was missing. Now looks aren't done to me—aren't *at* me—they're shared.

★ ★ ★

Efrem says he's afraid I'm going to leave him.

What a switch.

He says I'm different—that the change on my outside has brought a change to my inside—something has switched in me.

I tell him I'm still trying to grasp it myself—the actual switch. Have *I* changed, or has the world I'm walking around in changed—into an alternate reality or some kind of weird reflection-pool thing? A layer of gel, or gauze, like the thinnest onionskin, has been lifted, and the world beneath looks the same but behaves differently, because *I* appear different.

For instance, here—now—in my C-cup reality, I'm suddenly taken seriously. I can feel it—even with Ef. Like the eye-contact thing all over again—I only know I was missing it before because of its prevalence now. It's refreshing to be taken as a balanced package, rather than for boobs with a big mouth and thank-God brains, which is what I guess was happening. Ef's friend, Richard, who for some reason thinks in cartoons, said *before* that I was a cross between Little Annie Fanny and Charlotte Brontë (whatever that means or looks like). So what am I now?

I tell Efrem I feel like making some changes, but I don't think he's one of them. Now that he's responding to me so openly, I wonder out loud what he sees in me. I've never completely supported myself. I've never been out on my own.

★ ★ ★

I'm not allowed to jog yet or do sports or ride horses, but I can skate wearing my Jogbra. I'm warned to be careful, not to make wild motions, to steer clear of the wild motions of others, and no falling, please. Aggie skates guard, says if I lose my balance to grab on to her instead of bracing a fall on my own. She's acting more protective of me—says I'm beginning to seem like her little sister again, and she's been missing that.

"Really?" I ask her. I tell her, "Me, too."

We have picked back up meeting at the Boardwalk, rolling onto Sunday restaurant patios in shorts, in kneepads, in legwarmers, sparkly sweatshirts tied around our waists, to eat brunch while the coastal haze burns off, and we splurge on everything we know *we'll* burn off skating. After brunch, we Velcro on wrist-guards, and we skate up the Speedway and the Ocean Front bike path, to the Santa Monica Pier and back. Except now, when we roll past that one pavilion, my brown-bag bum doesn't say a thing.

INTERVIEW: T.J. MILLER

WHAT HAVE YOU LOST THE MOST SLEEP OVER IN YOUR LIFE?

T.J. Miller: I lost a lot of sleep filming *Yogi Bear* because of a number of things, but mostly it was the extreme stress of making a talking bear comedy and trying to make it the best possible piece of acting/cinema/comedy that I've ever been involved in. I didn't sleep much in New Zealand. Nightmarish dreamscapes of disparate forests with evil bears trying to thwart the happiness of millions of children plagued me endlessly.

DO YOU HAVE ANY ROUTINES OR REMEDIES FOR WHEN YOU CAN'T SLEEP?

T.J. Miller: I never have trouble sleeping. I always fall asleep whenever I lie down or sit in a seat, because I'm so tired all the time. I work a lot. Sometimes if I'm really tired and I haven't fallen asleep for a few minutes, I'll have an elderly Polish man sing to me while brushing my hair and, maybe if I have the money, I'll have his cousin, Yelmin play the spoons very softly.

WHERE'S THE STRANGEST PLACE YOU'VE EVER SLEPT??

T.J. Miller: Once I fell asleep on top of a sleep researcher. Crazy story, can't tell the whole thing legally, but basically, let's just say "HE DIDN'T CATCH A

WINK!" HAHAHAHAHAHA! Honestly though, his family was seriously affected and it was a pretty bad situation.

DO YOU HAVE ANY RECURRING DREAMS/NIGHTMARES OR THEMES THAT POP UP REGULARLY?

T.J. Miller: I'm always having nightmares about not being able to dream anymore.

COULD YOU TELL ME ABOUT A TIME WHEN YOU DID SOMETHING OUT OF CHARACTER WHILE SLEEP-DEPRIVED??

T.J. Miller: This is a good story actually: I came to Los Angeles in 2007 to film the pilot for *Carpoolers* and had never stayed or really been in L.A. I thought it would be funny (as I have occasion to do) to ONLY eat sushi, breakfast lunch and dinner. I was making a lot of money and I thought that was a pretty ridiculous thing to do and a good story to tell. But about day three, I started to have problems sleeping a little bit, and I started acting weird. I walked into a fire hydrant and smashed my car up pulling out of a garage. I didn't know what was going on. Later I found out that I was suffering maybe from mercury poisoning, and the lack of sleep plus that was making me a real weirdo and I was starting to go insane. Basically, the worst reason ever to lose sleep or run into a hydrant is eating sushi breakfast lunch and dinner. So that was my first Hollywood idiocy. For sure.

NIGHTTIME IN GIBBERISHTOWN

DAKOTA SEXTON

I'm twenty years old when people start to spill the beans that I talk in my sleep. I leave my studio apartment in the somewhat-hip neighborhood of Bucktown, in Chicago for a brownstone house a couple miles away—somewhere in-between the not-hip portion of Logan Square and

the even less hip neighborhood of Hermosa. Logan Square is notorious for becoming another new Wicker Park, the Bushwick to Brooklyn's Williamsburg. What notably resides near the corner of Fullerton and Springfield at the time I am twenty, however, are long stretches of marginally different liquor stores and laundromats, late-night taquerias, and a candy store with rainbow-colored letters that read, "Dulcelandia."

I immediately fall in love. I am even more in love with the idea of sharing an apartment with fifteen other individuals, a few rats, countless homeless traveler kids in their late teens and

twenties and a couple dozen mice. When I find out that none of my roommates shower frequently, I don't want to live anywhere else.

★ ★ ★

Depending on how much you sweat during the summer, the real funk probably doesn't start to linger for a couple of days or up to a week. Try not showering for a couple months and the funk in your house starts gaining additional notes, like a complex, nuanced perfume. The mice add charm as they scurry behind the stove as a burner comes on in the kitchen, or as they leave tiny

holes in the middle of everyone's collections of underwear, choose to leave even more miniature balls of poo along every wall, and make delicate scratching noises as I fall asleep at night.

The mold that's smelled yet never quite seen is considerably worse; not only is it the unknown culprit to the eternal question, "How could I be so tired today?" but also the source of stink in bedrooms, flooded landings, and a somewhat nauseating mixture of mildew and pee that seems to purvey any punk house bathroom where individuals don't actually flush the toilets. Our punk house is definitely that kind of punk house.

Yet I like it. And the less I shower, the more I feel at home. Besides the company of traveler kids and sometimes-unemployed roommates, our two-story apartment is also filled with early nineties films and Bollywood videos, and its countless bookshelves are lined with DIY gynecology zines and books by the likes of Murakami to Zizek. When I bike home from work, I alternate between blasting my personal anthem, "Punk Rock Girl," the new They Might Be Giants children's album, or a collection of indistinguishable hardcore punk music that probably has something to do with either feeling poor or living with crushing emotions.

I feel comfortable enough to pass out midday a couple hours after work in our first-floor living room. This is when it begins. I fall asleep on a couch, my mouth open and my arm hanging off the edge. On the first inexplicable night of note, my favorite barely-legal runaway roommate, Schroeder starts arranging sheets on top of a mattress between the couch I am asleep on and a sofa-sized futon next to our miniature TV. She rubs her face, crawls in between the sheets, and starts to lie down.

"Schro you can't do that…" I say, and sit up.

Schro looks over. My eyes are closed, my arms awkwardly arranged over my torso, and my mouth is open. She turns back toward the television.

"You can't do that. You gotta get the stick out of the bed." Schro looks back. My eyes are still closed. My mouth is still uncomfortably open. "You gotta—" I pause and motion toward the kitchen with a limp arm as Schro's face scrunches up at me, staring at my long eyelashes and my barely parted lips, before I shake myself, head and shoulders, and mumble, "Oh never mind. I'll do it myself tomorrow," and lie back down.

Schro doesn't. She lies awake, staring at the uneven white dots on the ceiling of the first floor, occasionally pausing to glance over at me. For the rest of the summer I sleep walk and soliloquize to myself, but much more publicly I also unintentionally try to hold my own in rational conversations about post-colonialism, mixing gibberish a relatively-coherent argument. It's charming because it's harmless.

A year later I am discovered hovering over the bedside of my roommate in Prague, clutching a bright orange pair of scissors with my eyes closed.

There is no way to explain this.

I feel slightly more worried in Amsterdam when I stay with a twenty-six year old graphic designer named Bart who might or might not be a distant Dutch cousin.

I fall asleep on the floor of his bedroom while he sleeps on the elevated mezzanine level high above. I fall asleep between midnight and dawn the first night, I am suddenly, uncomfortably, aware that I am standing at the foot of his bed beyond a flight of steps, breathing hard and heavily and hoping that in the morning this will somehow transform into a very funny story that I can tell. At the breakfast table I watch Bart wait for espresso to boil in a tiny rusted pot on the stove. The espresso begins to boil just as one of his bald roommates sits down wearing only a towel and holding a cup of chamomile tea. Bart turns to mention that he did hear me in the night—trying to practice my Dutch. I not only spoke the equivalent of Dutch baby talk, I had even chimed in to correct myself; the Dutch word for "thank you," *dank u wel,* is actually pronounced "dank oo vell," not apparently, as I originally mumbled it, "dank well."

★ ★ ★

By the time that I arrive in Belgium about a week and a half later, I feel like honesty should probably be the best policy. At least after a couple of nights. After three nights on the living room floor of a mild-mannered couch-surfing host named Steven, I roll up my sleeping bag and fold the futon mattress beneath it with the intention of spilling my own beans. Someone who offers me a drink around midnight my first night in town, but then proceeds to hand me a glass of cold milk, not booze—probably deserves to know the truth about my sleep talking.

"So, how did you sleep?" I ask Steven as soon as he exits his bedroom and begins to head toward the kitchen. "I hope…um, well, I have to say, I kind of talk in my sleep," I say before he can answer, clutching my rolled sleeping bag.

Steven, already standing in between the doors of the refrigerator in the kitchen before I finish, stands still for a moment.

"You know, it takes an awful lot to surprise a Belgian," he says suddenly, milk carton in hand as he moves out from behind the refrigerator and closes its doors. "Ryan has night terrors," he adds, then motions toward the other bedroom in the apartment and smiles. I open my mouth and bite my lip. His smile grows. In my dreams, I know we would run toward each other and make out at this moment. I tell my deepest and darkest sleep-talking secrets, and he slams the refrigerator door, pausing for a moment before he says, "Darling, I don't give a damn," and smiles. In one intense moment, the milk carton falls from his hands and I throw my sleeping bag across the room and we run toward each other, the look on my face mirroring the look on his face, and we make love and it is absolutely amazing.

★ ★ ★

I fly home to Chicago a couple weeks later, back to a bedroom without windows in a three-bedroom apartment overlooking the grassy north edge of Humboldt Park. The apartment is almost a return to the squat I lived in on the so-called outskirts of Logan Square—dirty, yet now decorated with a feminine touch obvious in the swaths of dried lavender in our bathroom to the miniature bouquets of flowers on every windowsill. Instead of the cases of the dumpstered Odwalla that counted as a main food source, the new refrigerator is stocked with Schro's gourmet picks from his job at Whole Foods or the farmer's market finds of our spunky roommate Reagan. Our other roommate, Naomi, also contributes bits of Yiddish, gossip about north-side punk skins, and packages of kosher fake cheeses and meats.

I throw myself at a light fixture in my bedroom within a month, struggling to get the decorative glass cover off so that I can get to the light bulb inside it in time to escape a Poe-esque death scenario in which the walls of my already small and windowless bedroom have begun to close in, beckoning death, moments before Reagan runs in—not because she's angry, but because she imagined that someone finally managed to break into our ill-secured first-floor apartment and that I am risking life and limb to try to beat him up. I listen to her from my lofted bed, still clutching the light bulb in my

hand. The light fixture hangs helplessly by its wires, its screws already pulled directly out of the wall. White flecks of ceiling fall onto my arm. Reagan hugs her arms together and assures me that if I ever want to sleep next to her in the hallway between my bedroom and our back door, there will always be room.

I should be able to realize that no matter what obnoxious nightmares I have to try to overcome in the middle of the night, there will be always be someone willing to coax me back to sleep.

But I don't. I take a bus from New York's Port Authority terminal to a small county seat known as Honesdale in the foothills of the Poconos Mountains of Pennsylvania, hastily preparing in my seat for an internship interview at a yoga magazine published on the grounds of a retreat center. Instead of paying more attention to whether or not I'm dressed appropriately for the interview, I focus on how scared I am that someone will hear me shouting loudly in my sleep and that I will not be given the internship I need to graduate from college.

That doesn't happen. Or, rather—losing the internship doesn't happen. At breakfast someone informs me that she had thought someone else was with me in my room. When I explain my situation, she only says that it must be uncomfortable having such publicly loud dreams.

★ ★ ★

In a world where someone is turned on by my sleep talking, I can only dream that I'd also be the Clark Kent of sleep-active super heroes. I'd take on the assumed name, *The Sleepwalking Susan*. Posters would be wheat-pasted to city walls that portray me as a pint-sized superstar in my fearsome, nighttime lingerie, clutching ninja throwing stars behind a teddy bear. Giant, diagonal, yellow headlines would declare, "Fear the might of *The* Sleepwalking Susan! Her nighttime terrors have *fangs*!" Only while wearing spandex lingerie would I feel comfortable with the source of my power, however; stuck within a cockeyed universe that featured other super heroes with explosive, embarrassing farts for super powers, or maybe villains whose greatest feats most days only amounted to training other people's dogs how to pee on command.

Somehow—like Superman's fatal link to Kryptonite—sleep talking still remains something to feel uncomfortable about. If Batman ever spent time worrying about whether or not chicks would actually think his obsession with bats was cool, I spend inordinate amounts of time worrying about my own sleep-related peculiarities. Yet I am the mayor of gibberish town. I should be proud. Dystopian futures filled with lackluster, ripped-off *Poe* scenarios, robots who create robots to take over other robots who don't like good smells, or other constant cutthroat conflicts throughout the world so difficult that half the surviving human population merely becomes retired ninja heroes on Medicaid—should always, I can only hope will only—also include my serious bouts of sleep conversation, each one as bizarrely, perversely weird as the last.

SUPERHEROES DREAMING

WILLIAM HUGHES

Batman sleeps upside down. His friends think he's just really committed to the theme, but only he knows his terrible secret: he is a sleepwalker, and he is terrified that one day he'll wake up to find everything he's ever loved lying in a sleep-karate-chopped pile on the ground.

Wonder Woman doesn't sleep with stuffed animals anymore. She used to, but then her boyfriend made fun of her about it. She's still kind of mad at him about that, but she's also mad at herself. She's Wonder Woman, damn it. She shouldn't care what Jeff thinks.

Green Lantern sleeps on a bed of green energy formed from his VERY WILL. His roommates have asked him to stop, because it's really bright and now they can't sleep. They also want him to stop drinking their milk. Green Lantern doesn't care. Green Lantern is too cool to care.

Spider-man always puts a lump of webbing down on the bed, right before he goes to sleep. He claims it is for lumbar support, but really, he just likes the smell. It reminds him of his Spider-mom and Spider-dad.

Superman doesn't sleep, but he makes the bed every day, as soon as Lois gets out. If he doesn't make the bed, he feels like something terrible will happen. Lois tells him he needs therapy, but he just waves her off and grumpily reads Internet.

Wolverine sleeps outside on an air mattress. Every morning he wakes up by popping the air mattress with his claws, and then has some coffee. Then he goes to the air mattress store. He is in love with the lady who works there.

The Flash sleeps for 1/1000th of a second every five minutes. He dreams about turtles with low whispering voices and terrified eyes. They've been whispering something to him for the last 20 years. By the time he understands the message, it'll be far too late.

The Hulk is doing a sleep lab experiment this week. He keeps fidgeting with the EKGs and demanding juice from the puny sleep lab people. He is worried he has an apnea.

Wonder Woman's boyfriend Jeff sleeps just fine, thank you very much. Very fine indeed, yesiree bob. Jeff is an asshole.

Aquaman sleeps wherever he wants. Why not? He's King of the Oceans. He just tunes his fish telepathy to the frequency of jellyfish and slowly drifts to sleep. Bobbing in the waves, they whisper soothing jellythoughts as he slips away into dreaming.

Robin has nightmares. Every night he watches people die, people he could have saved. He hasn't told anyone. Sometimes he wets the bed from fear, but he cleans the sheets before Alfred can see.

He's supposed to be stronger than this.

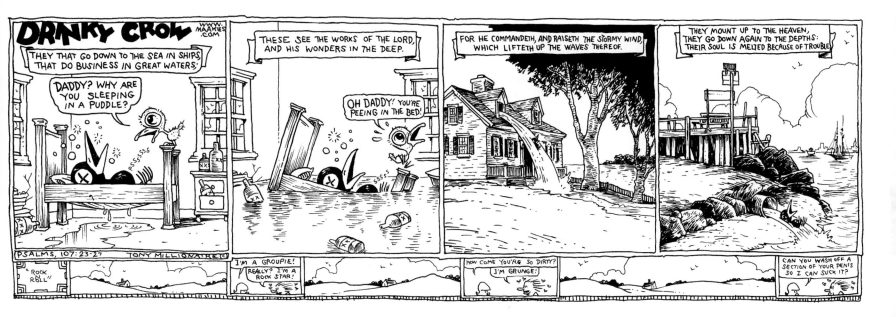

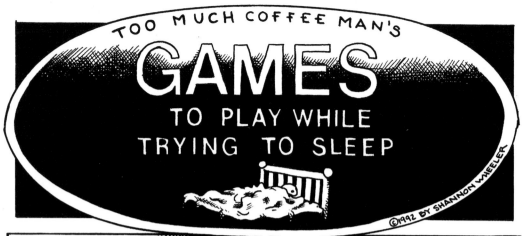

TOO MUCH COFFEE MAN'S
GAMES
TO PLAY WHILE TRYING TO SLEEP

©1992 BY SHANNON WHEELER

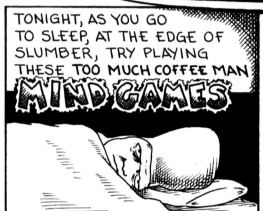

TONIGHT, AS YOU GO TO SLEEP, AT THE EDGE OF SLUMBER, TRY PLAYING THESE **TOO MUCH COFFEE MAN** MIND GAMES

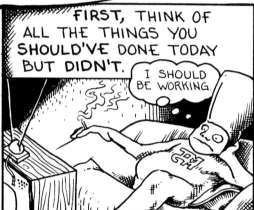

FIRST, THINK OF ALL THE THINGS YOU SHOULD'VE DONE TODAY BUT DIDN'T.

I SHOULD BE WORKING.

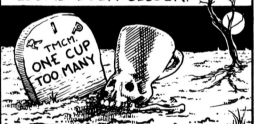

NOW THINK ABOUT YOUR **LIFE** AND HOW MUCH **TIME** YOU'VE **WASTED** AS THE YAWNING CHASM OF **DEATH** LOOMS EVER CLOSER.

TMCM. ONE CUP TOO MANY

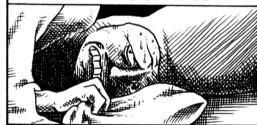

BUT **DYING** WILL ONLY ACT AS A **COMFORT** AS YOUR **MIND** TRAVELS BACK TO **RE-LIVE** ALL THE **HUMILIATING** INCIDENTS OF CHILDHOOD.

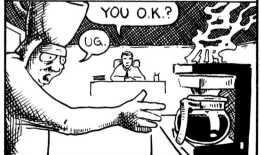

THINK ABOUT HOW MISERABLE YOU'LL BE IF YOU **DON'T** MANAGE TO GET **SOME** SLEEP!

YOU O.K.?

UG.

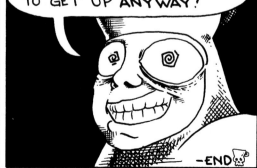

BUT REMEMBER: IN ONLY A FEW HOURS YOU'LL **HAVE** TO GET UP **ANYWAY!**

—END

28.

WHAT SHOULD I wear tomorrow, JEANS, T-SHIRT, sure, what COLOR, does it matter, Not sure

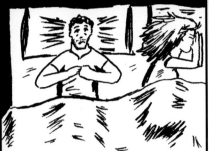

DID we PAY the MORTGAGE, yes, maybe,

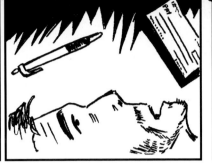

OKAY, but WHY is the TEXTING portion so HIGH, is there an UNLIMITED PLAN, and why do I need to TEXT anyone

Couldn't I CALL or email,

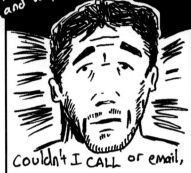

YES, I could TWITTER, though what is that REALLY, and WHY would someone DO IT...

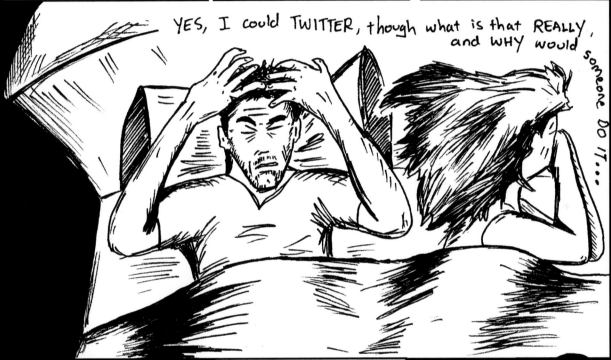

does anyone but LIZ care what I'm up to all the time, every second of the day, WHY IS THAT FUN, maybe I am too old to get it...

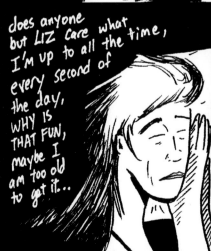

MONICA, man she's smoking

oh. hey Keith.

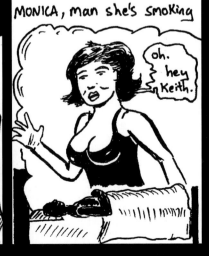

AND the LOCKS, DID we LOCK the DOOR, LAST NIGHT, yes, TONIGHT, maybe, but BOTH LOCKS, can't say, should I check, NO, yes, NO, NO, probably, maybe, is that MOANING? yes it is, weird, and SHIT, is the ALARM set, yes, yes, CHECK, CASHED, CHECK AGAIN, COOL, and the DOOR, just IGNORE IT

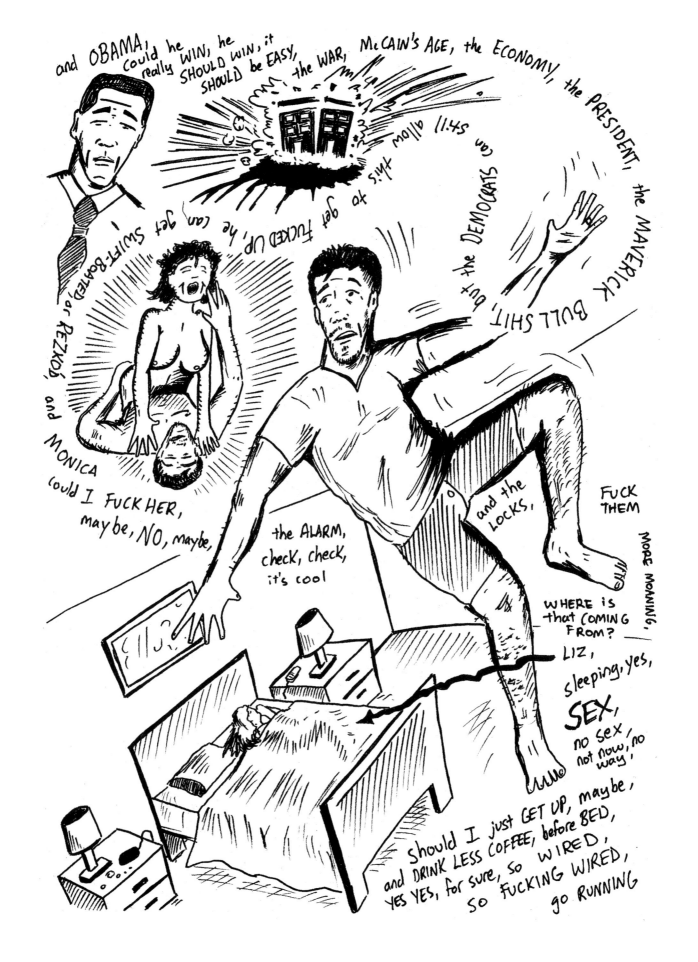

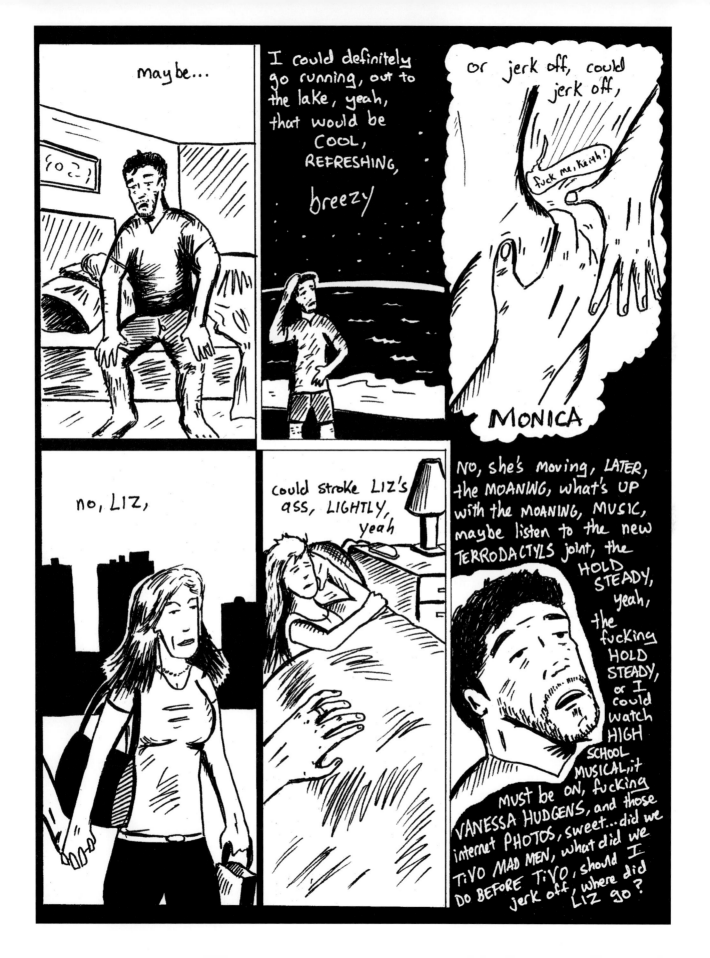

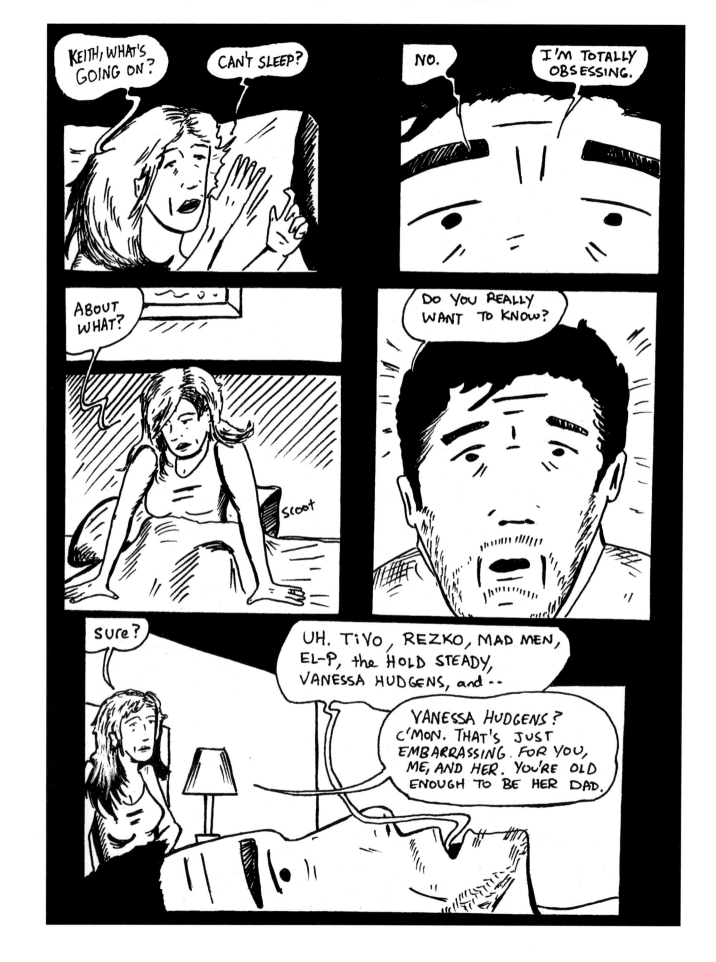

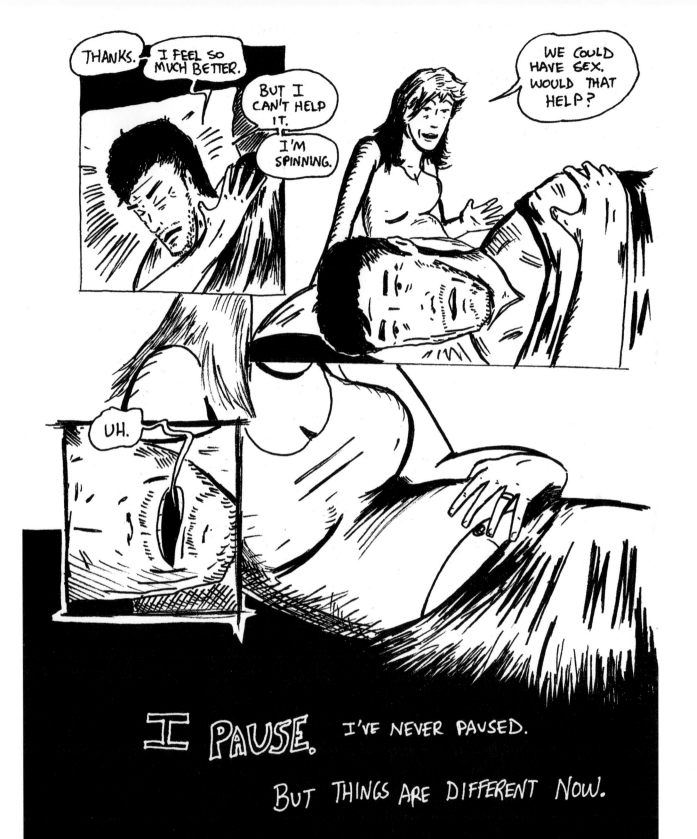

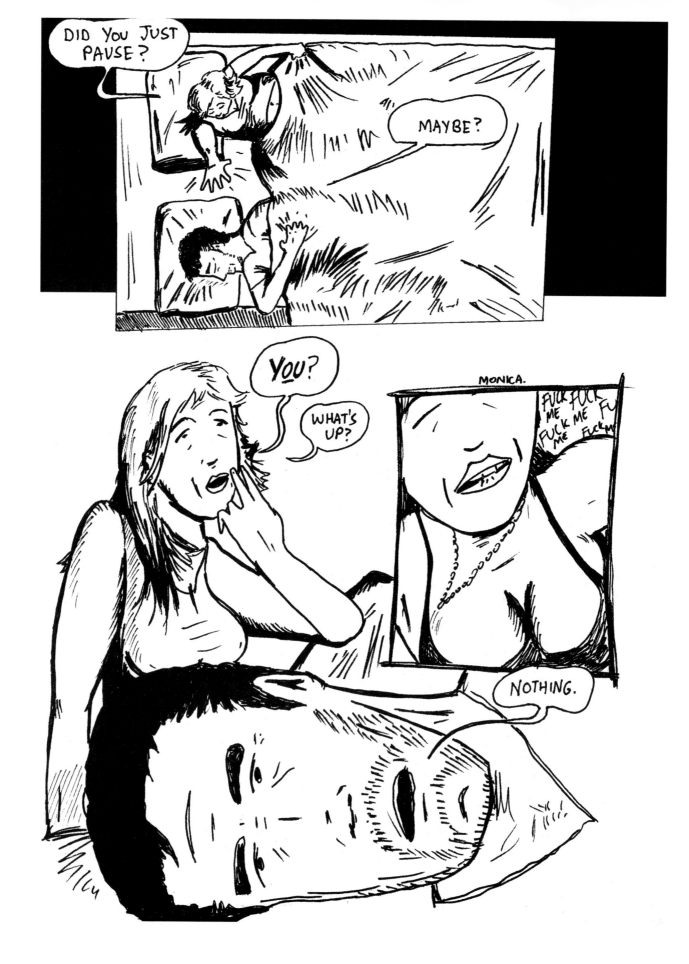

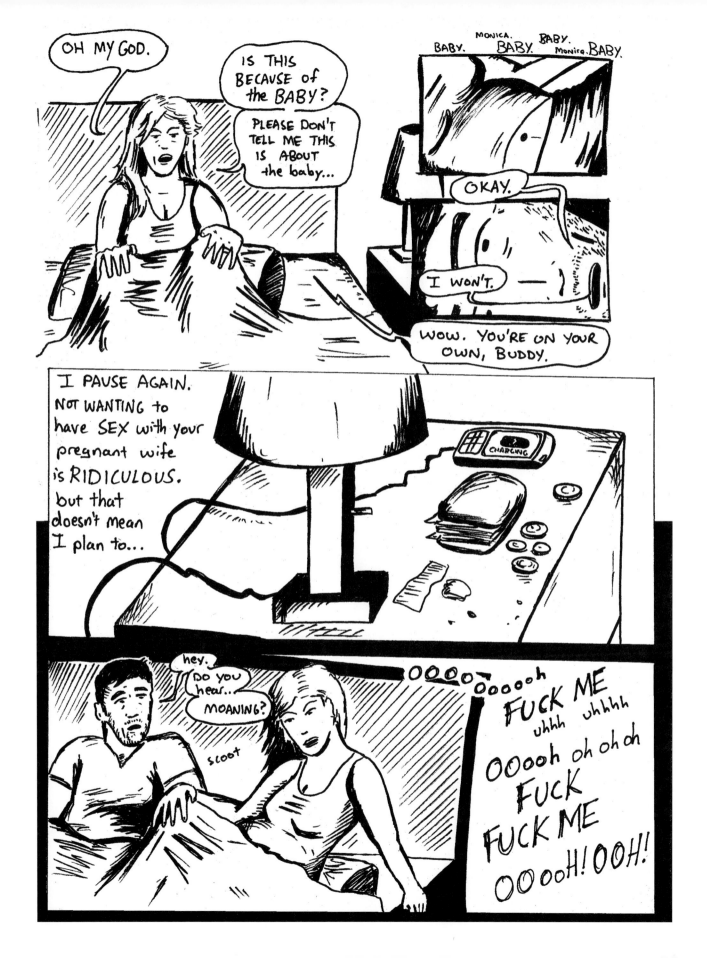

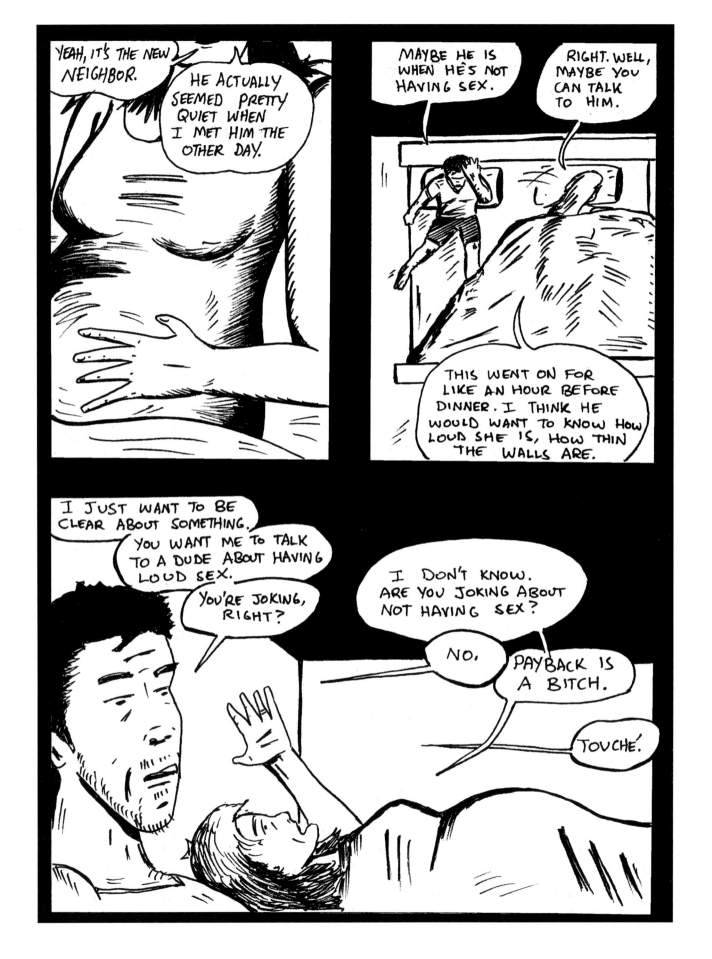

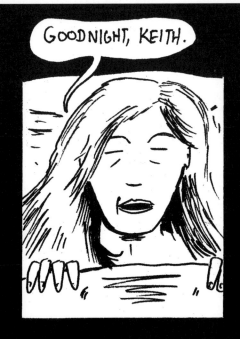

GOODNIGHT, KEITH.

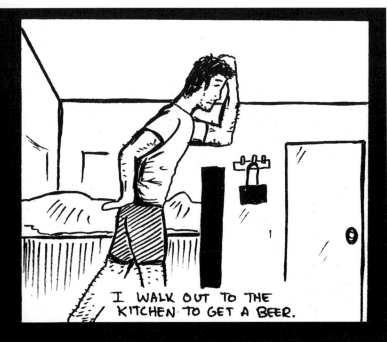

I WALK OUT TO THE KITCHEN TO GET A BEER.

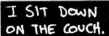

I SIT DOWN ON THE COUCH.

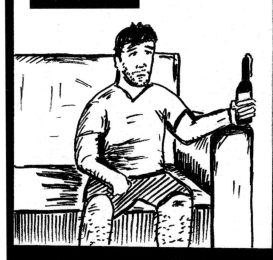

I PUT ON THE HOLD STEADY AND "STUCK BETWEEN STATIONS" STARTS UP.

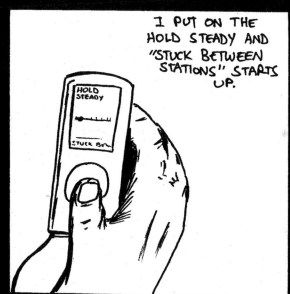

MY HEAD IS STILL SPINNING, MY THOUGHTS AND COMPULSIONS ON THE KIND OF ENDLESS LOOP THAT EVEN THE HOLD STEADY CAN'T DERAIL. THIS BABY THING IS NOT GOOD AND THERE WILL BE NO SLEEP TONIGHT.

I FINISH MY BEER.
I LOOK FOR MY RUNNING SHOES.

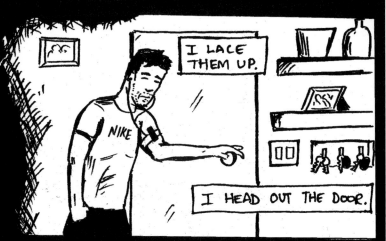

I LACE THEM UP.

I HEAD OUT THE DOOR.

The Do's & Don'ts Of Taking A Nap

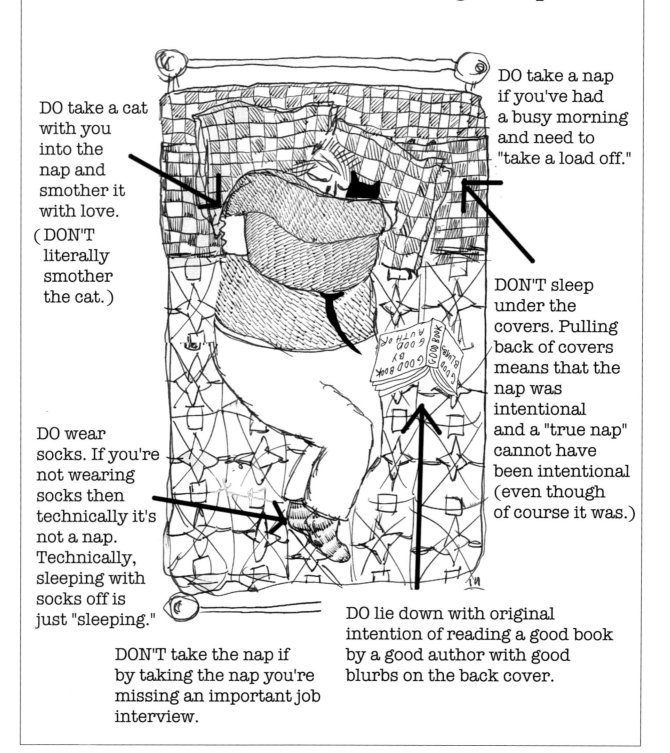

DO take a cat with you into the nap and smother it with love. (DON'T literally smother the cat.)

DO take a nap if you've had a busy morning and need to "take a load off."

DON'T sleep under the covers. Pulling back of covers means that the nap was intentional and a "true nap" cannot have been intentional (even though of course it was.)

DO wear socks. If you're not wearing socks then technically it's not a nap. Technically, sleeping with socks off is just "sleeping."

DON'T take the nap if by taking the nap you're missing an important job interview.

DO lie down with original intention of reading a good book by a good author with good blurbs on the back cover.

LET ME SLEEP ON IT

a comic by Kenny Keil

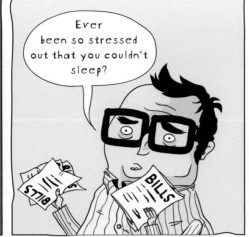

Ever been so stressed out that you couldn't sleep?

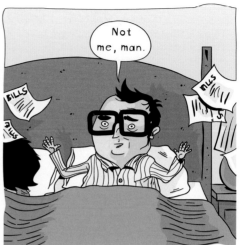

Not me, man.

For some reason, stress has always had the opposite effect on me— it actually makes me sleepy!

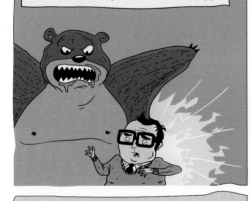

"Fight or flight?" Are those really my only options? Personally I find that many of life's problems can be solved (or at least postponed) by simply lapsing out of consciousness

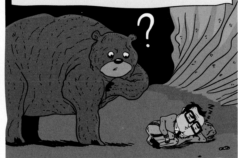

Take air travel for example. Isn't it one of the most gut wrenching, powerless experiences a human can endure? Well, I wouldn't know, because I'm not staying awake long enough to find out.

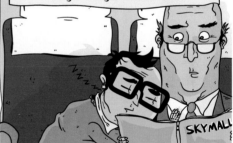

(Aside from when the snack cart rolls around, that is.)

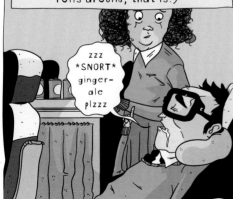

I mean, what am I gonna do in case of an actual emergency, take the wheel? Might as well go out comfortably.

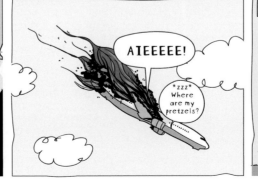

Believe it or not, this condition can actually have its advantages on occasion. Like that one time back in '97, at the high school state track meet

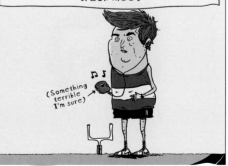

I had a tendency to get so stress-sleepy before a big race that I'd wind up exhausted long before I even got to the starting line. And that day was no exception...

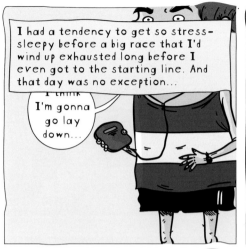

I think I'm gonna go lay down...

So this time, instead of stretching, warming up, etc. I went and found a nice, quiet grassy area not too far from the track and took a nap...

Half an hour later I was at the starting line, feeling relaxed, refreshed and ready to go!

I ran those two miles with a zen-like calm unlike anything I'd ever felt before. Not only did I win the race, but I also set a new state record!

THANK YOU!

You're too kind!

BULLY FOR YOU, OLD CHAP!

waiiit a minute...

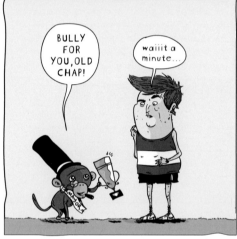

True, I'd accidentally slept through the race and the whole thing turned out to be a dream. But so what?

The point is, that feeling of accomplishment has stayed with me to this very day

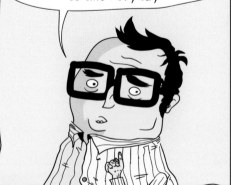

So the next time life gets to be too much for you, just sleep it off! Trust me, you'll be glad you did.

CLICK

G'night!

ZZZ

FZZZAT

the end

It seems like everybody else in the world spends all their time trying to find someone to share the rest of their lives with.

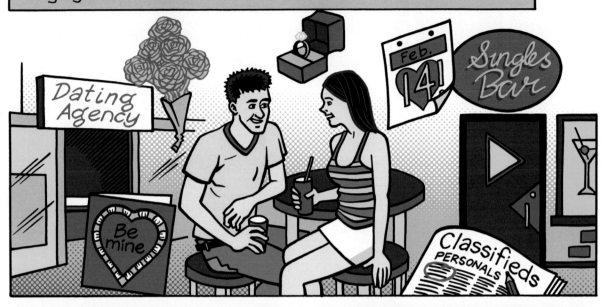

Me? I go to sleep every night wondering if I'll ever know what it's like...

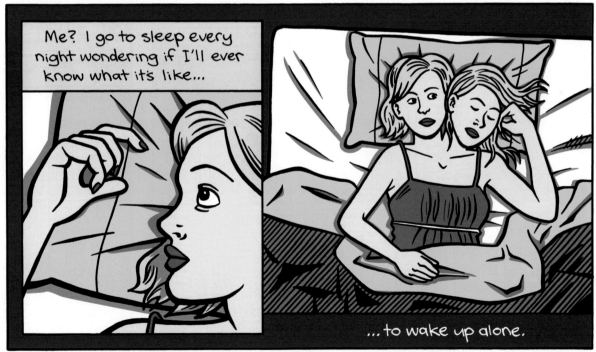

... to wake up alone.

...better than one? Words + pictures: OWEN HEITMANN

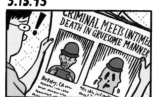

Erika's Dreams

© DAVID HEATLEY & ERIKA CLOWES

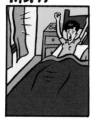
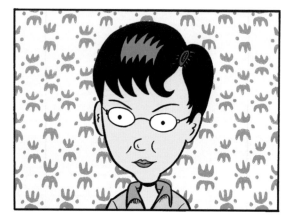
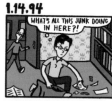
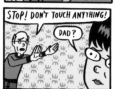
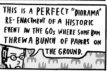
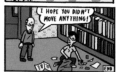
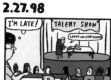

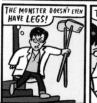

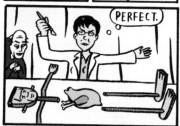
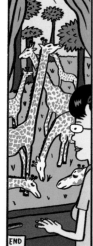
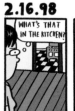
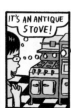
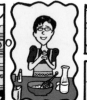

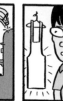
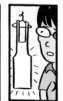
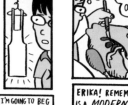
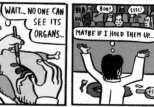
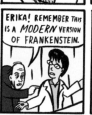
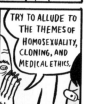
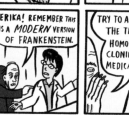
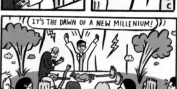

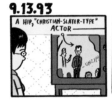

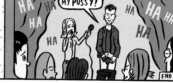

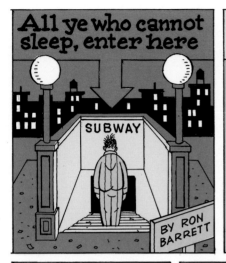

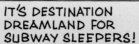

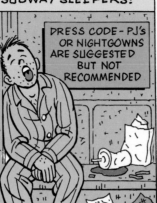

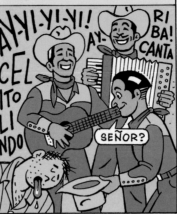

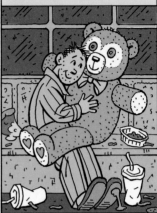

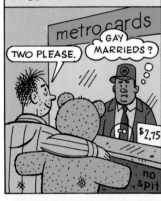

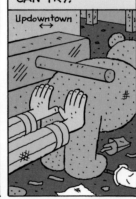

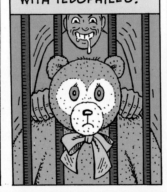

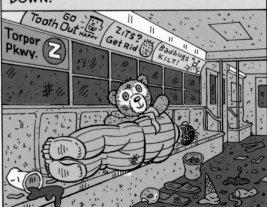

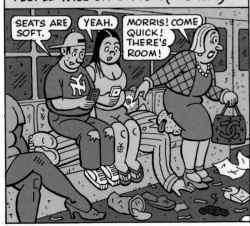

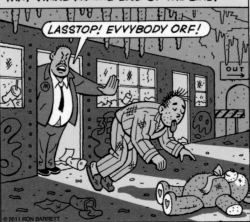

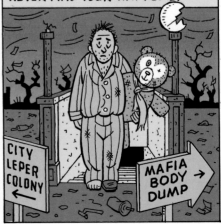

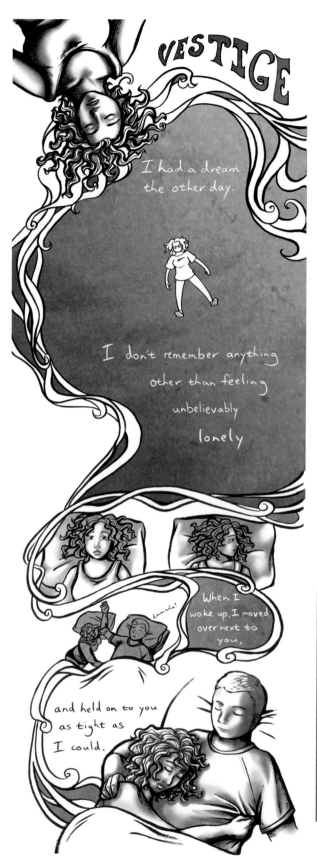

VESTIGE

I had a dream the other day.

I don't remember anything other than feeling unbelievably lonely

When I woke up, I moved over next to you,

and held on to you as tight as I could.

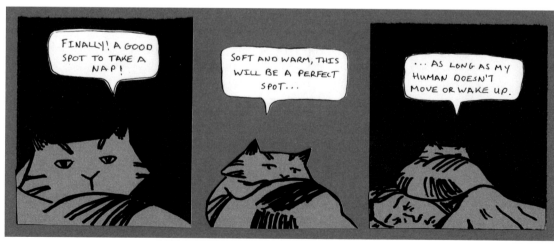

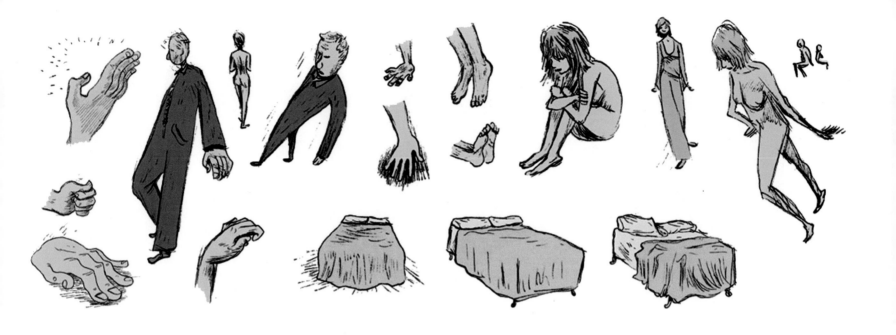

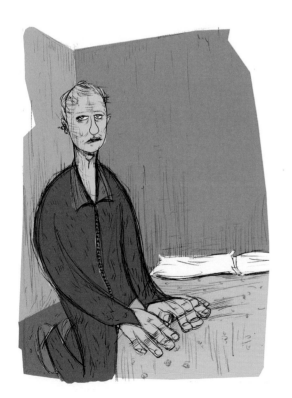
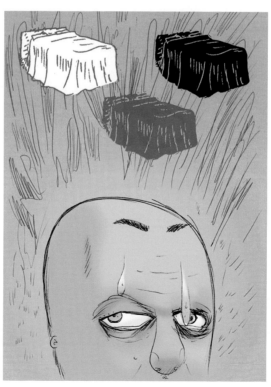
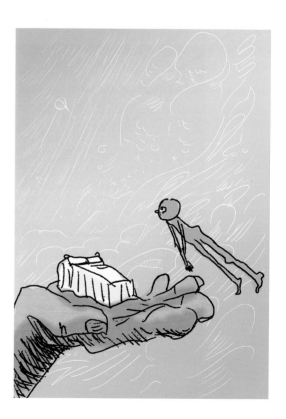

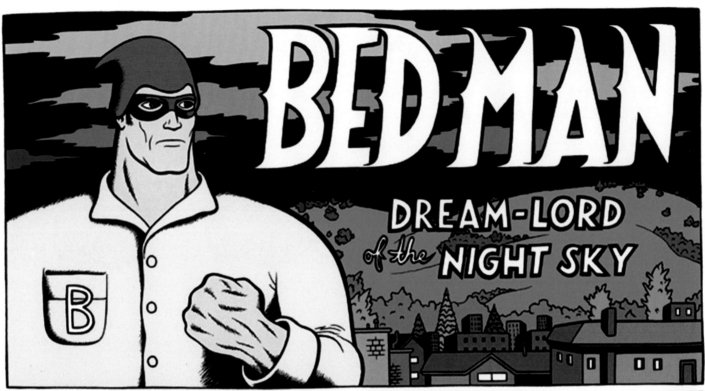

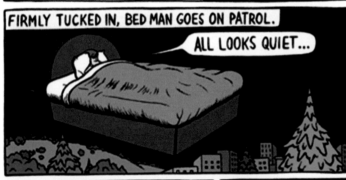

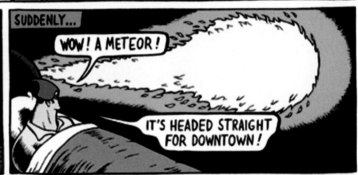

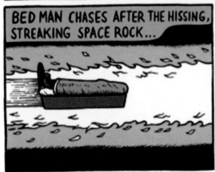

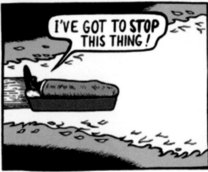

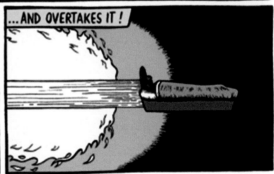

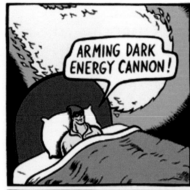

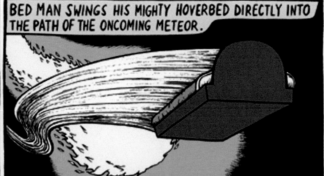

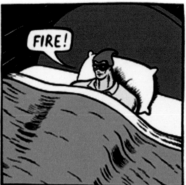

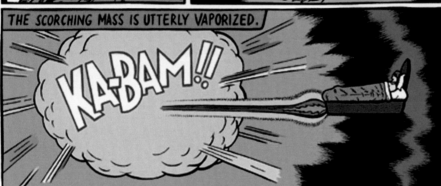

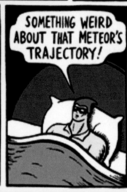

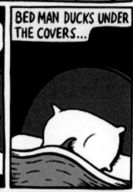

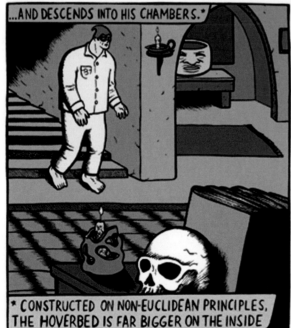

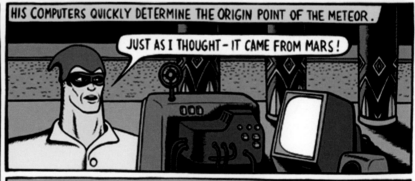

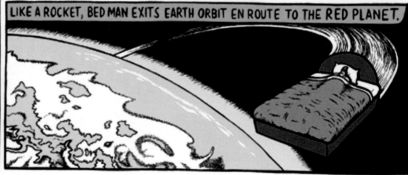

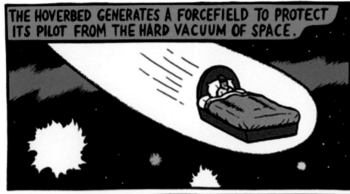

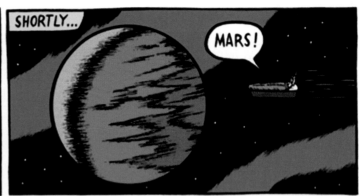

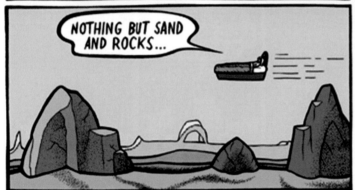

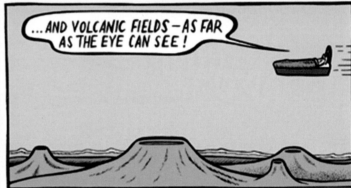

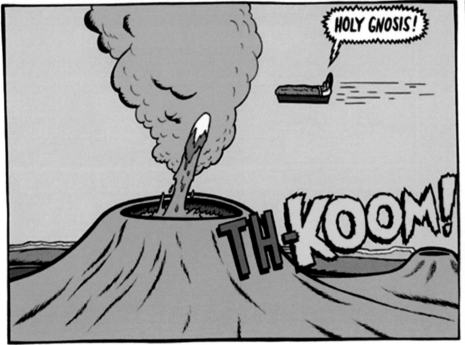

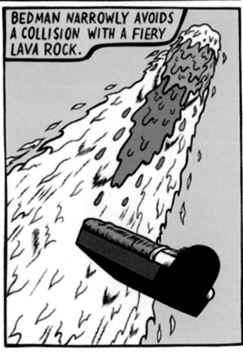

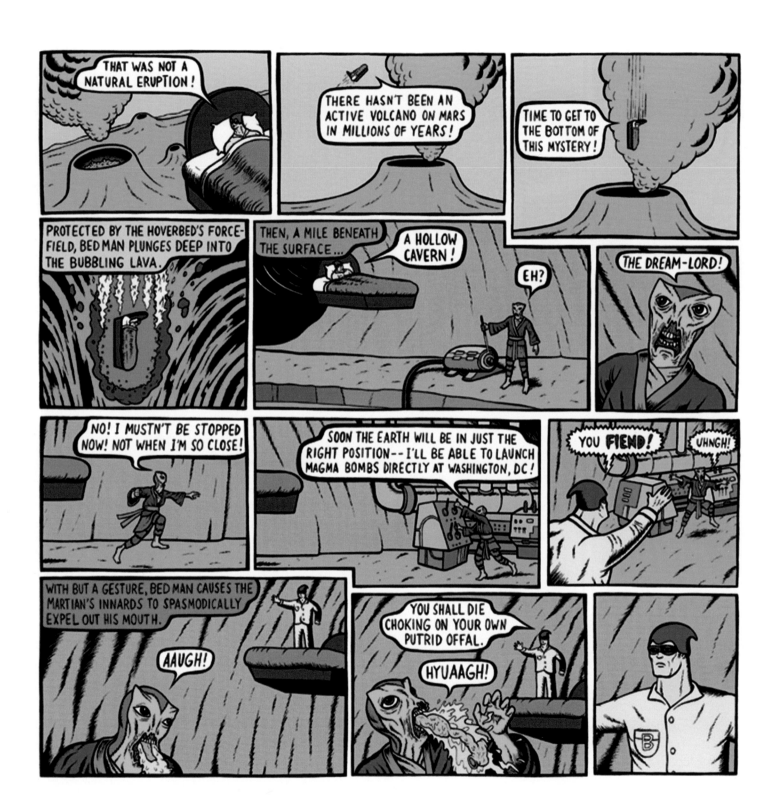

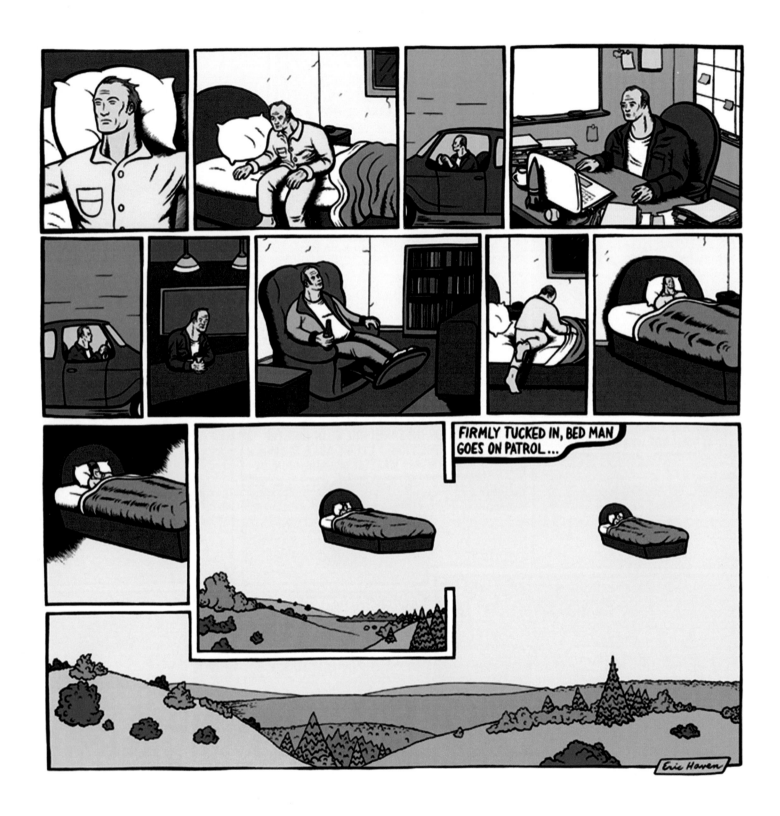

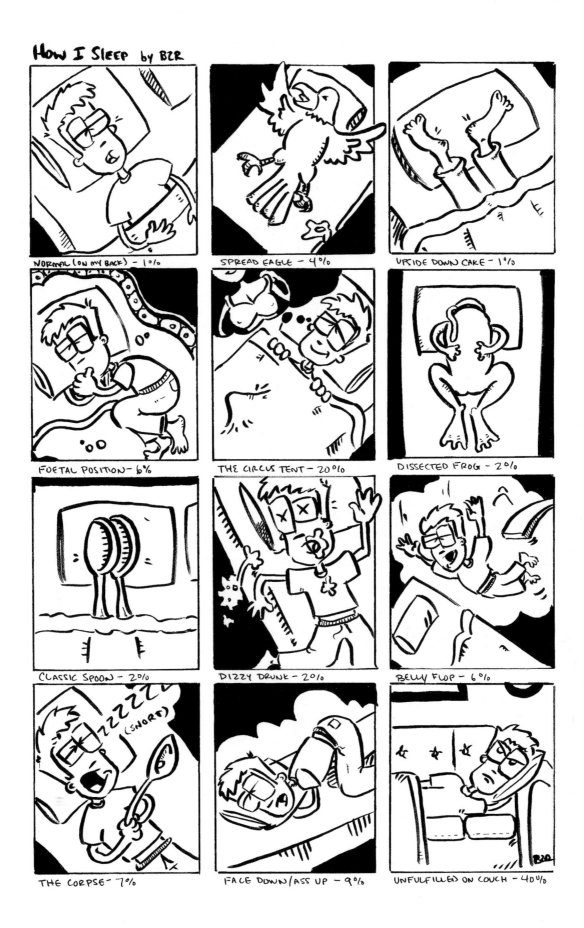

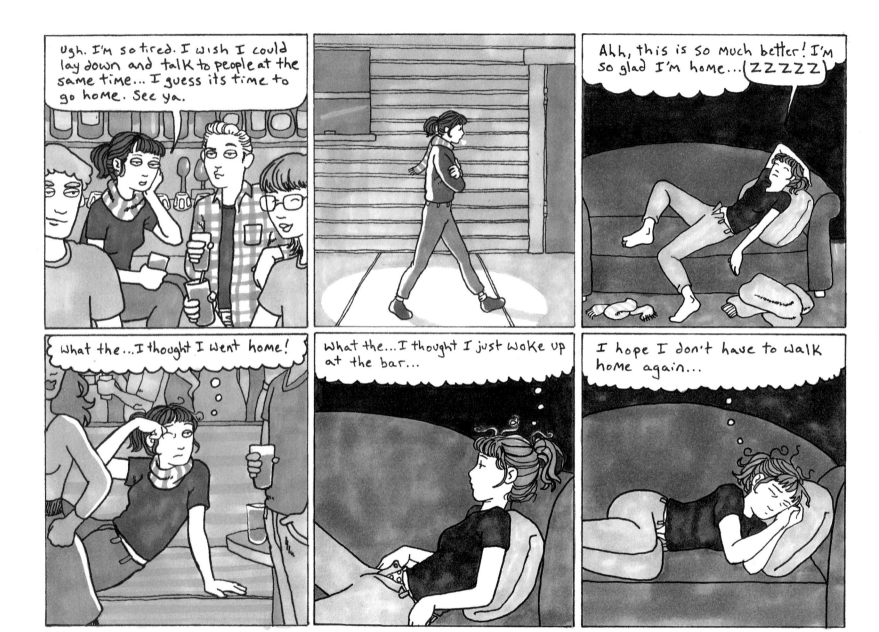

melon
by Cynthia Hawkins

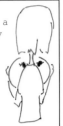

Her face appeared on a white, shiny plate and stayed that way.

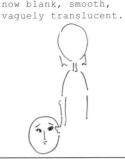

The place where her face had been was now blank, smooth, vaguely translucent.

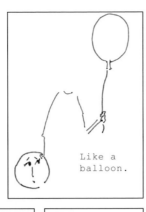

Like a balloon.

She tried

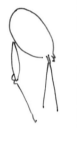

communing

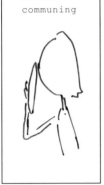

with

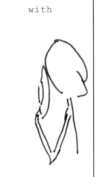

the plate.

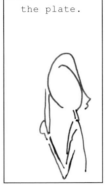

It didn't work.

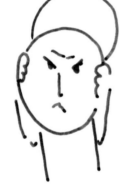

She was afraid of dishwashers.

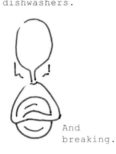

And breaking.

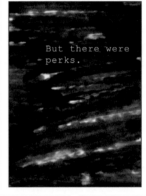

But there were perks.

She could be slid under a sofa

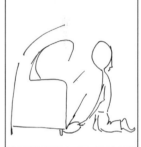

to look for spare change and paperclips.

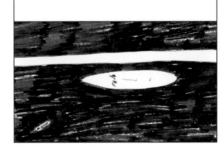

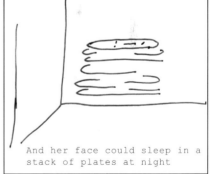

And her face could sleep in a stack of plates at night

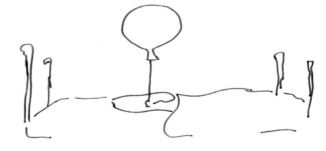

while the rest of her dreamed of eating cantaloupe.

THE EARLIEST DREAM I CAN REMEMBER OCCURED WHEN I WAS ABOUT FOUR.

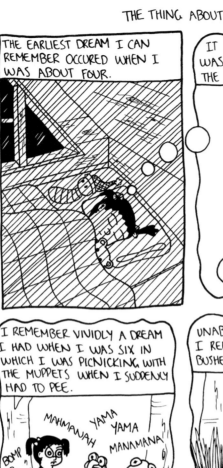

IT INVOLVED A LARGE, SESAME STREET LOOKING WORM WHO WAS TRYING TO MAKE ME SOLVE MATH PROBLEMS, DESPITE THE FACT THAT I DIDN'T KNOW HOW.

I'M TRYING! I'M TRYING! BUT IT'S JUST THAT I DON'T KNOW HOW!

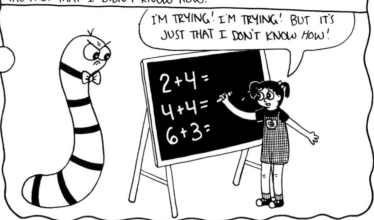

I REMEMBER VIVIDLY A DREAM I HAD WHEN I WAS SIX IN WHICH I WAS PICNICKING WITH THE MUPPETS WHEN I SUDDENLY HAD TO PEE.

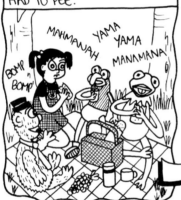

UNABLE TO FIND A BATHROOM, I RELIEVED MYSELF IN THE BUSHES BEHIND A ROCK.

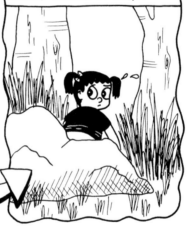

UNFORTUNATELY, THE ACTION CARRIED OVER INTO REAL LIFE.

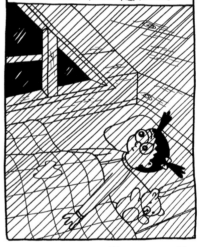

EVER SINCE, WHENEVER I SEE THE MUPPETS, I'M STRUCK WITH A SUDDEN, YET MERCIFULLY FLEETING, URGE TO URINATE.

AH, A BEAR IN ITS NATURAL HABITAT... A STUDEBAKER

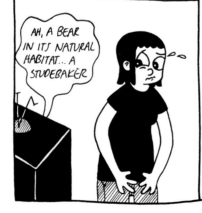

THE REST OF MY CHILDHOOD DREAMS WERE FAIRLY ORDINARY.

...AND THEN I WAS IN THE LIVING-ROOM BUT IT WASN'T OUR LIVINGROOM BUT IT WAS, YA KNOW? AND THE DUCK FROM U.S. ACRES WAS THERE WITH A BOX OF BABY SALAMANDERS! I WAS LIKE, WHAAAAT!

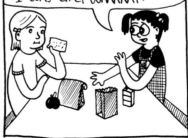

THE ONLY REOCCURING DREAM I HAD WAS ABOUT BEING LOST IN A JELLYFISH AQUARIUM, WHICH HAD HAPPENED ONCE IN REAL LIFE.

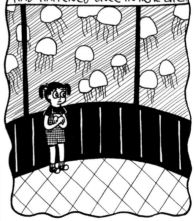

IN MY TEEN YEARS, I HAD FREQUENT HOME INVASION NIGHTMARES. (I SUSPECT THIS WAS A DIRECT EFFECT OF TEEN SLASHER FILMS)

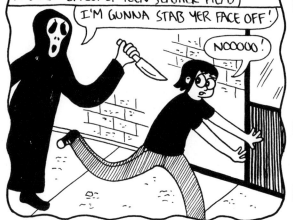

I'M GUNNA STAB YER FACE OFF!

NOOOOO!

DURING THE RARE, LUCID DREAM, I ALWAYS DEFAULTED TO A SPECIFIC AGENDA.

OH! I'M DREAMING! I HAVE TO FIND SOMEONE TO MAKE OUT WITH STAT!

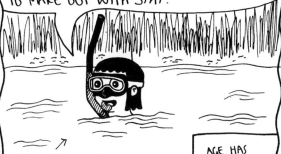

SNORKLING IN THE NILE, A FREQUENT DREAM THEME

AGE HAS NOT SWAYED THIS MISSION

FOR MANY YEARS, NIGHTMARES AND/OR INSOMNIA REPEATEDLY FOILED MY ATTEMPTS TO QUIT DRINKING.

FUCK SOBRIETY AND GETTING MY LIFE BACK TOGETHER, I JUST WANNA SLEEP

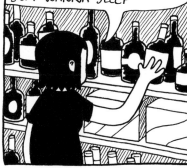

I TRIED OVER THE COUNTER AND PRESCRIPTION SLEEPING PILLS, BUT THEY ALWAYS HAD THE ADVERSE EFFECT.

WHY AM I AWAKE RIGHT NOW? IT DEFIES HUMAN BIOLOGY!

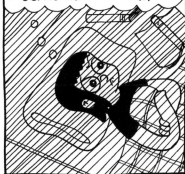

I DIDN'T UNDERSTAND THAT AFTER YEARS OF DRINKING MYSELF TO SLEEP, MY BODY CHEMISTRY WAS ALTERED TO THE POINT WHERE IT DIDN'T KNOW HOW TO SHUT DOWN WITHOUT ALCOHOL.

NNNG... I'M GONNA BE AWAKE FOR THE REST OF MY LIFE!

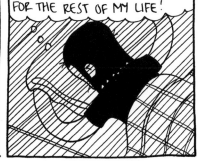

IN MY LATE TEENS, I WENT THROUGH A BRIEF PERIOD OF FASCINATION WITH DICTATORS, SOME OF WHOM TENDED TO POP INTO MY DREAMS AT THE MOST INAPPROPRIATE TIMES.

FIDEL?! I THOUGHT YOU WERE AXL ROSE!

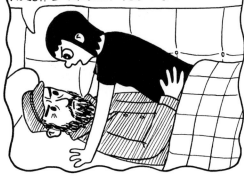

MY DREAM LIFE TOOK A TURN FOR THE WORST IN MY MID 20'S AFTER MY FIRST REAL ATTEMPT TO QUIT DRINKING. I BEGAN TO HAVE HORRIFYING, EPIC NIGHTMARES IN WHICH I WAS CONSTANTLY TRYING TO SURVIVE THE APOCALYPSE WITHOUT ANY SHOES ON.

AAAH! IT'S ALL SHATTERED GLASS AND SPLINTERED BONES! I'LL NEVER MAKE IT OUT ALIVE

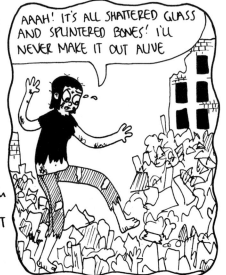

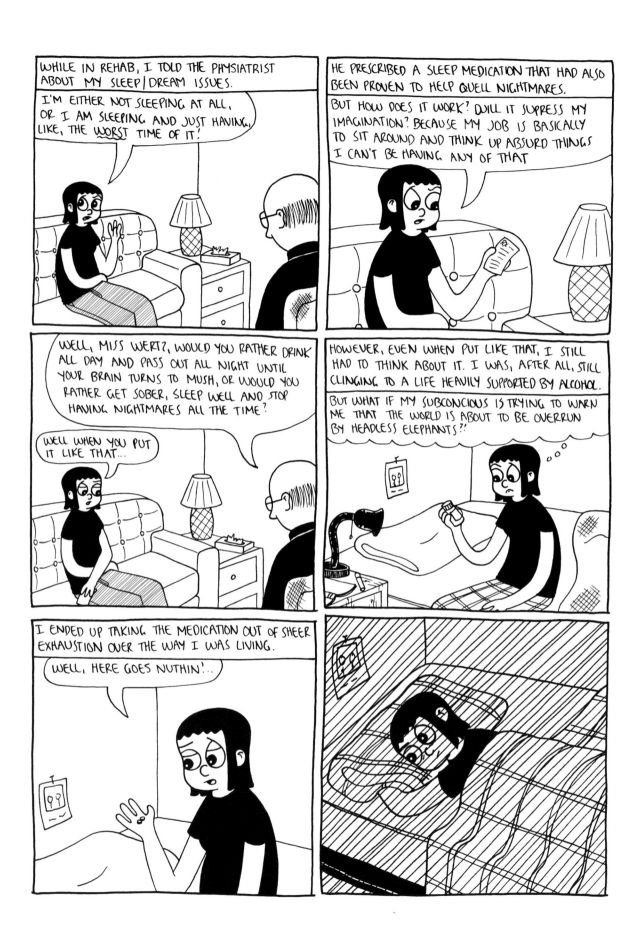

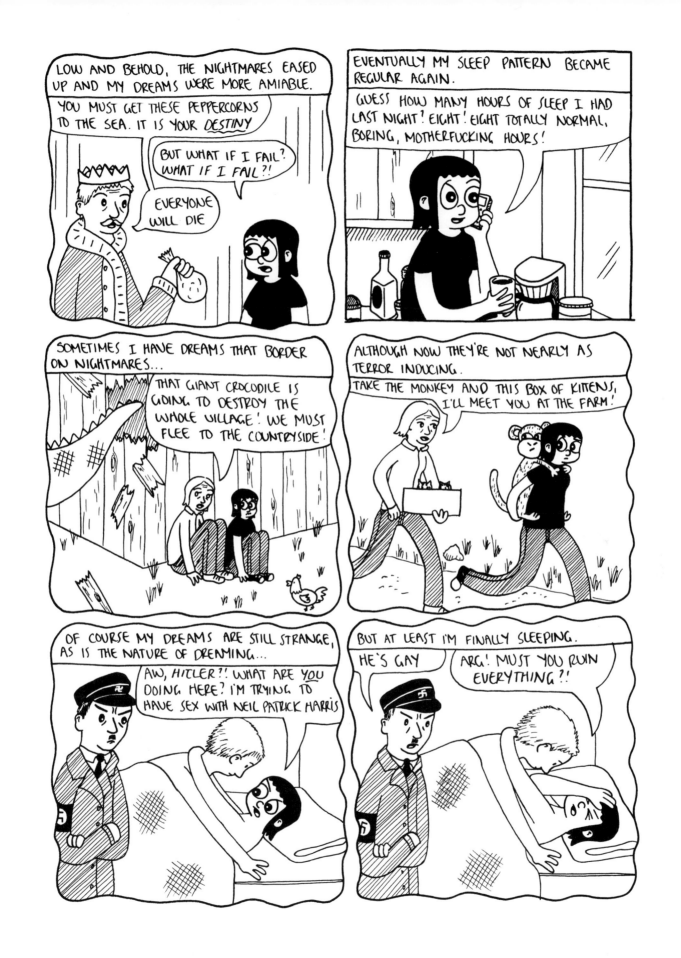

SLOW WAVE

by Melissa Gawlowski and Jesse Reklaw

MY MOTHER WAS SPRINKLING POISON INTO OUR MORNING OATMEAL.

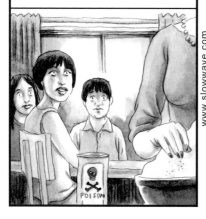

SHE TOLD US NOT TO WORRY, BECAUSE SHE'D MIXED IT WITH BROWN SUGAR TO TASTE NICE. AND ANYWAY, JESUS TOLD HER TO DO IT.

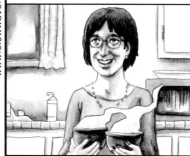

I LOOKED OVER AND JESUS WAS WATCHING THE PROCEEDINGS, CHECKING OUR NAMES OFF ON A CLIPBOARD.

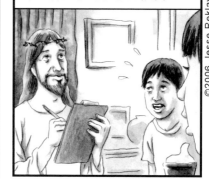

I WAS SCARED TO DIE, BUT IT WORKED OUT BECAUSE ONCE I GOT TO HEAVEN, I RECEIVED A PLAQUE.

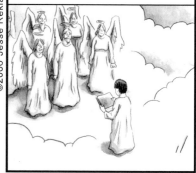

©2006 Jesse Reklaw

SLOW WAVE

by Kris Seeman and Jesse Reklaw

I AM RIDING A WINGED UNICORN THROUGH MISTY MOUNTAIN TOPS AS FAR AS THE EYE CAN SEE.

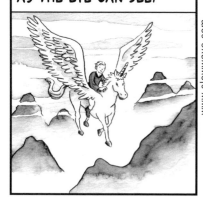

I LAND AT EACH ONE, DISMOUNT, THEN FIND A CAVE AND EXPLORE IT. I AM SEARCHING FOR THE WORLD'S ONLY BATHROOM.

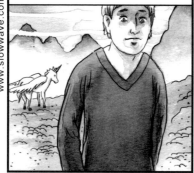

I HAVE SEARCHED ABOUT TEN CAVES WITHOUT SUCCESS. AT THE NEXT ONE, I COME UPON A SMALL WARRIOR GNOME.

The commode you seek is a long way from here.

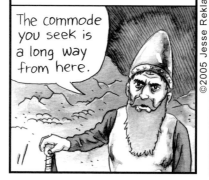

HE ISN'T SURE ABOUT ITS PRECISE LOCATION BUT POINTS IN THE GENERAL DIRECTION. I THANK HIM AND DEPART ON MY NEVER-ENDING JOURNEY.

Good luck!

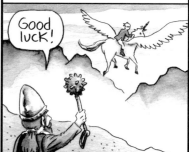

©2005 Jesse Reklaw

SLOW WAVE

by Keith Ridgway and Jesse Reklaw

I WAS SITTING AT THE EDGE OF A SWIMMING POOL, WHEN I NOTICED SOME ROADS AND FIELDS ON MY LEFT SHOULDER.

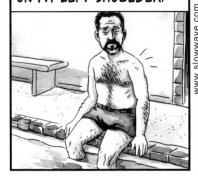

LOOKING CLOSER, I SAW TINY CITIES RISING FROM THE SKIN OF MY SHOULDER, WITH ROADS, FIELDS, AND THOUSANDS OF PEOPLE.

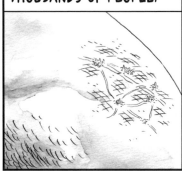

IT LOOKED LIKE ONE ARMY WAS HEADING TOWARDS ANOTHER, ABOUT TO LAUNCH INTO A BATTLE.

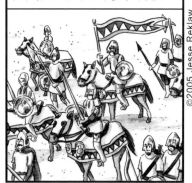

I THOUGHT THAT WAS YUCKY, SO I PUSHED OFF THE SIDE OF THE POOL AND INTO THE WATER TO DROWN THEM ALL.

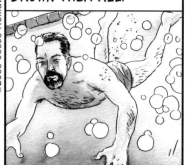

©2005 Jesse Reklaw

www.slowwave.com

SLOW WAVE

by Cynthia Walker and Jesse Reklaw

THERE WAS A KNOCK AT THE DOOR. IT WAS THE GRIM REAPER.

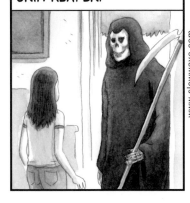

HE WAS SELLING POORLY DRAWN AND OUTDATED WORLD ATLASES. WE ARGUED OVER THE SHAPE OF THE PACIFIC OCEAN.

It doesn't look anything like this!

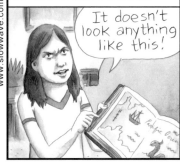

HE STARTED TO CRY. I FELT REALLY GUILTY, SO I DECIDED TO HELP HIM ON HIS SALES TOUR.

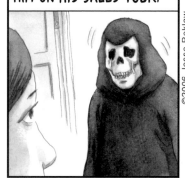

BECAUSE WHO NEEDS TO KNOW THE TRUE DIMENSIONS OF THE PACIFIC ANYWAY? MOSTLY PEOPLE JUST FLY OVER IT.

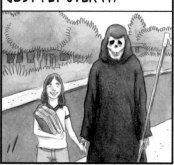

©2006 Jesse Reklaw

www.slowwave.com

SLOW WAVE

by Alan Wolfe and Jesse Reklaw

PEOPLE AT WORK ARE GETTING CASH BONUSES, BUT I RECEIVE A DEAD BIRD IN A ZIPLOC BAG FULL OF WATER.

Way to go! *Lucky!*

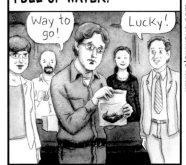

A CO-WORKER TELLS ME THIS IS THE BEST TYPE OF BONUS. ONE DAY THE BIRD WILL COME TO LIFE AND GIVE ME CAREER ADVICE.

Donald Trump had one just before he made it big.

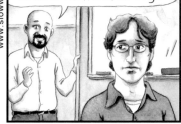

I LEAVE IT ON TOP OF MY COMPUTER. SOMETIMES ITS EYES OPEN AND STARE AT ME. THIS MAKES ME REALLY UNCOMFORTABLE.

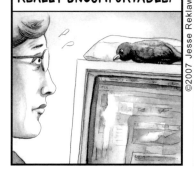

I TRY THROWING IT AWAY, BUT THE CLEANER BRINGS IT BACK.

You can't throw away the bonus bird! Bill Gates had one just before...

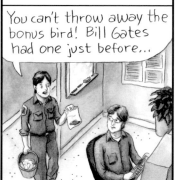

©2007 Jesse Reklaw

www.slowwave.com

I guess you could say I'm one of those people who "sleep to dream". As entertaining as dreams can be sometimes, I'm more intrigued with the fact that there is no definite exlpanation of what they are, and why we have them.

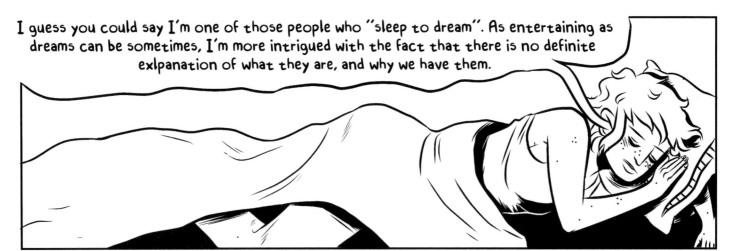

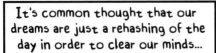
It's common thought that our dreams are just a rehashing of the day in order to clear our minds...

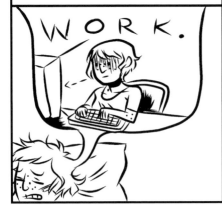

But what about those dreams you just can't explain? Ones that can't possibly be linked to the waking world. What about those?

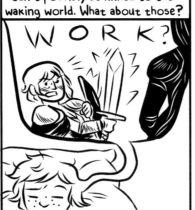

I've often wondered if there really is such a thing as a dream world...

Have you ever wondered why you dreamt of a certain person? What if maybe it's because they were dreaming about you?

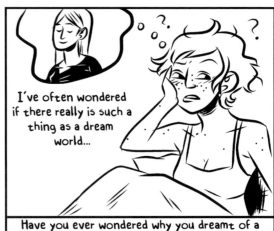

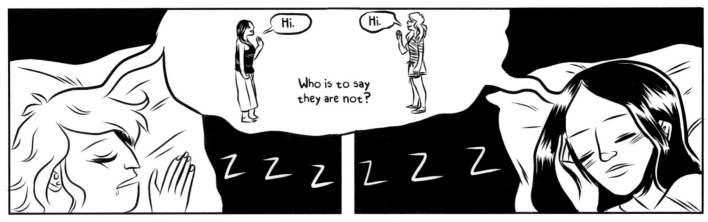

Hi.

Hi.

Who is to say they are not?

It's common to dream of people you see on a daily basis. Not only friends or family, but coworkers or classmates could find their way into your dreamspace.

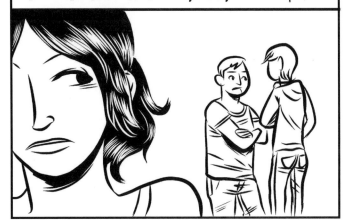

In fact, there was a girl who found herself frequently dreaming of a boy she barely knew. Almost every night he made an appearance one way or another.

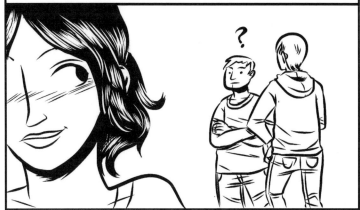

Over time, and as the dreams continued, she actually started to fall in love with him.

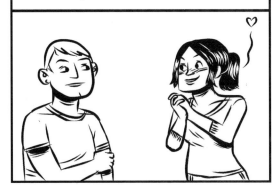

However, she found that he was aboslutely nothing like how she dreamt him to be.

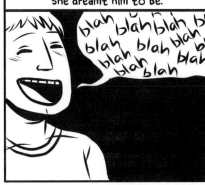

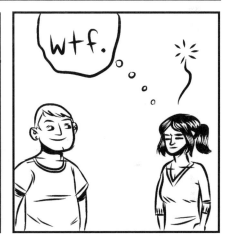

wtf.

It's pretty amazing how strong our subconscious is. Based on dreams alone, this girl fell in love with someone she had not known otherwise.

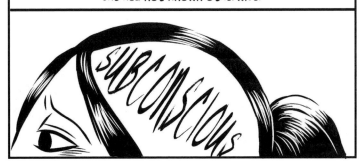

But what about strangers? Have you ever had a dream about someone you've never seen before?

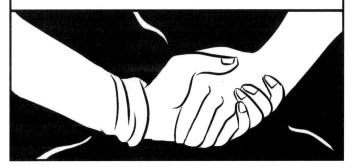

A few months ago I had a dream that I came across a stranded car in the snow with a boy trapped inside.

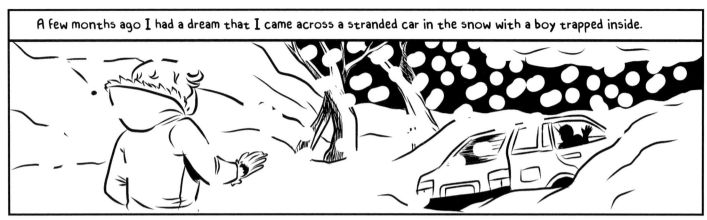

With some force I was able to pry open the door, free him...

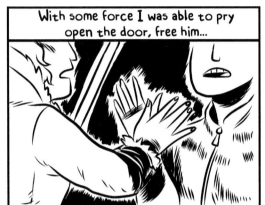

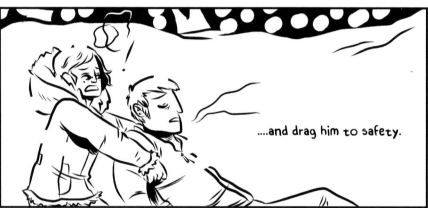

....and drag him to safety.

I didn't really think too much of the dream...

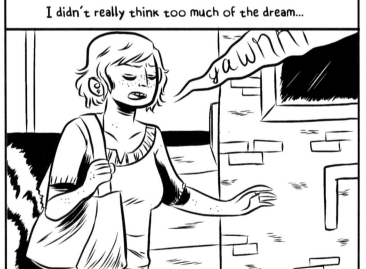

yawnnn

...until that boy showed up at my workplace.

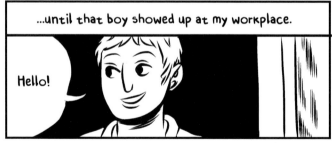

Hello!

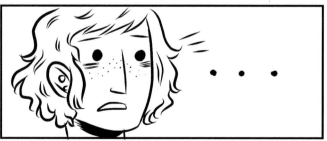

. . .

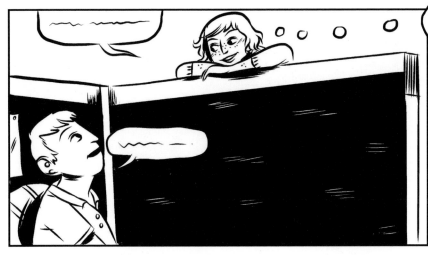

Maybe he just has a familiar face?

This is more than likely the case. It's possible that he reminded me of someone I just couldn't place at the time (still can't).

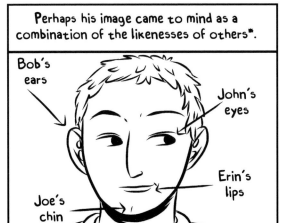

Perhaps his image came to mind as a combination of the likenesses of others*.

Bob's ears

John's eyes

Erin's lips

Joe's chin

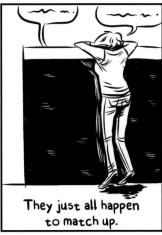

They just all happen to match up.

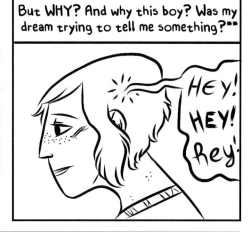

But WHY? And why this boy? Was my dream trying to tell me something?**

HEY! HEY! Hey!

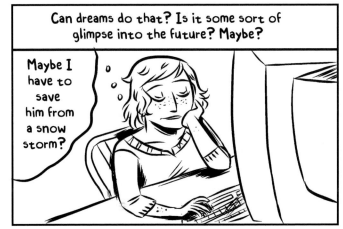

Can dreams do that? Is it some sort of glimpse into the future? Maybe?

Maybe I have to save him from a snow storm?

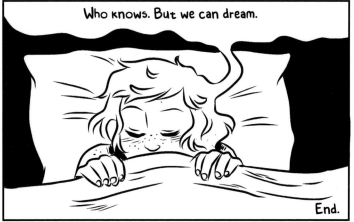

Who knows. But we can dream.

End.

*These are not real people.
** The dream was completely PLATONIC, as was the brief friendship with dream boy.

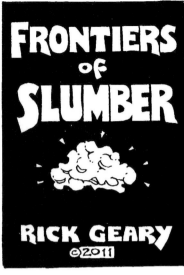

FRONTIERS of SLUMBER

RICK GEARY
©2011

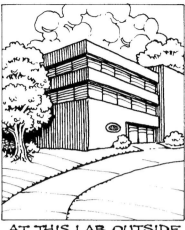

AT THIS LAB OUTSIDE BAYONNE, OUR TEAM LEADS THE WORLD...

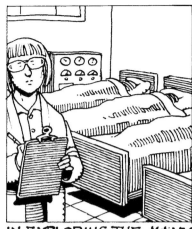

IN EXPLORING THE MANY MYSTERIES OF SLEEP.

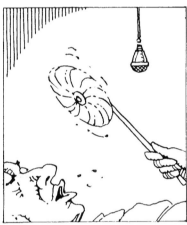

CAN SNORING BE HARNESSED AS A SOURCE OF ENERGY?

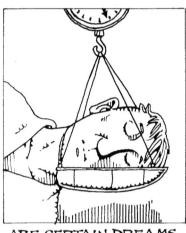

ARE CERTAIN DREAMS "HEAVIER" THAN OTHERS?

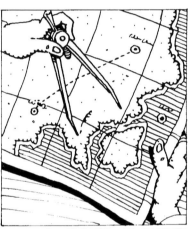

CAN A NIGHT OF SLEEP BE "MAPPED" AS IF A TERRITORY APART?

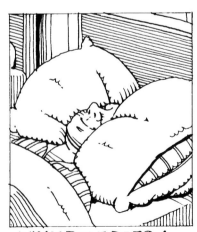

WHAT ROLE DOES A GOOD PILLOW PLAY?

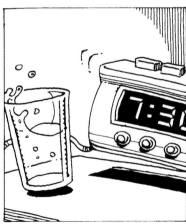

AND "WAKING UP" BRINGS ITS OWN SET OF PROBLEMS.

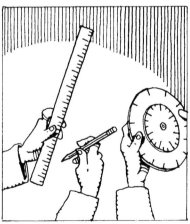

OUR BIGGEST CHALLENGE WAS TO MARK THE EXACT MOMENT WHEN SLEEP BEGINS.

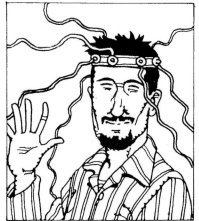

I WAS THE DESIGNATED GUINEA PIG FOR THAT ONE.

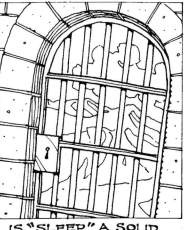

IS "SLEEP" A SOLID BOUNDARY, WITH, FOR INSTANCE, A HEAVY IRON GATE?

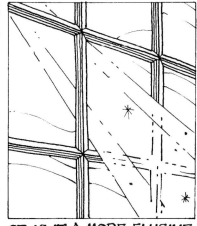

OR IS IT A MORE ELUSIVE TRANSITION, LIKE A RAY OF LIGHT THROUGH GLASS?

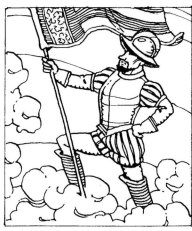

I SAW MYSELF AS A TRAILBLAZER... A "CONQUISTADOR OF SLUMBER."

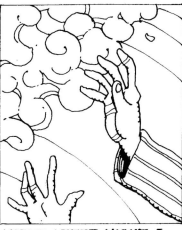

NIGHT AFTER NIGHT I TRIED TO REACH THE THRESHOLD...

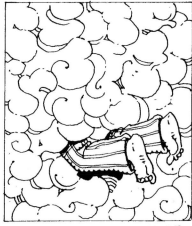

BUT TOO SOON I DRIFTED INTO UNCONSCIOUSNESS.

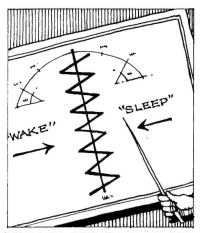

THEN IT OCCURRED TO ME: WHY NOT APPROACH IT FROM THE OTHER SIDE?

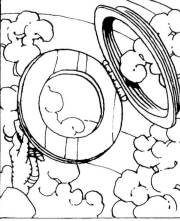

IT WORKED! THERE'S THE PORTAL AT LAST!

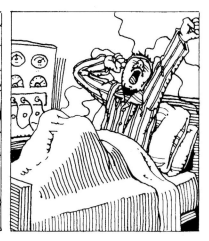

ANOTHER BREAKTHROUGH!

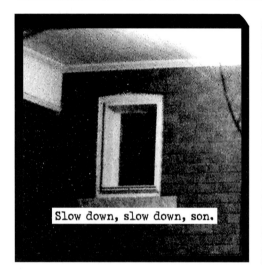

Slow down, slow down, son.

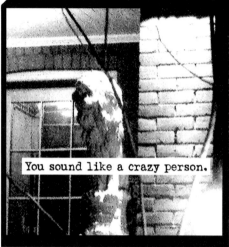

You sound like a crazy person.

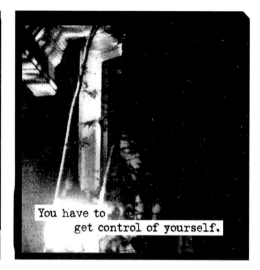

You have to get control of yourself.

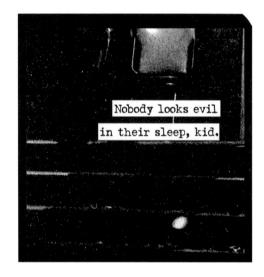

Nobody looks evil in their sleep, kid.

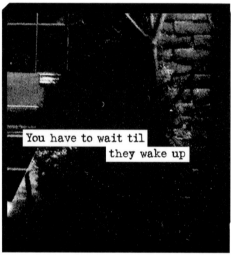

You have to wait til they wake up

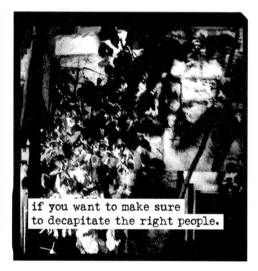

if you want to make sure to decapitate the right people.

BED SQUAD COP by Ron Barrett

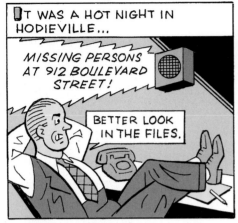

IT WAS A HOT NIGHT IN HODIEVILLE...

MISSING PERSONS AT 912 BOULEVARD STREET!

BETTER LOOK IN THE FILES.

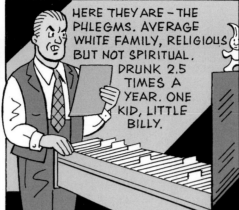

HERE THEY ARE – THE PHLEGMS. AVERAGE WHITE FAMILY, RELIGIOUS BUT NOT SPIRITUAL. DRUNK 2.5 TIMES A YEAR. ONE KID, LITTLE BILLY.

I WENT OUT TO 912 BOULEVARD STREET TO INVESTIGATE...

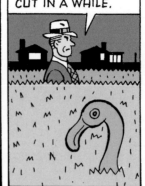

LAWN HASN'T BEEN CUT IN A WHILE.

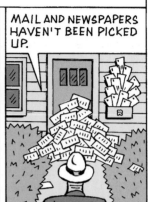

MAIL AND NEWSPAPERS HAVEN'T BEEN PICKED UP.

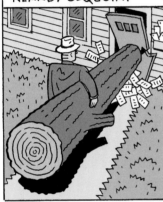

I DECIDED TO ENTER FORCIBLY, USING A NEARBY SEQUOIA.

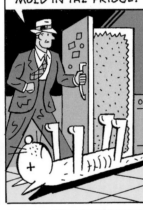

HMMM... CAT HASN'T BEEN FED. THERE'S MOLD IN THE FRIDGE.

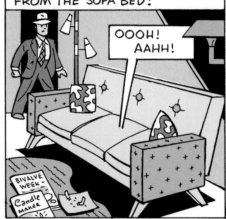

THEN I HEARD IT— THE SOUND FROM THE SOFA BED!

OOOH! AAHH!

BIVALVE WEEK –
Candle maker

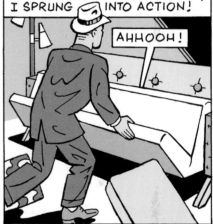

TOSSING THE CUSHIONS ASIDE, I SPRUNG INTO ACTION!

AHHOOH!

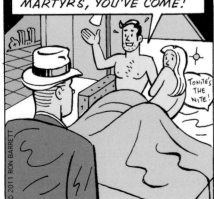

THE JAWS OF THE BED DISGORGED THE PHLEGMS!

THANK GOD AND THE BLESSED BLOOD OF ALL THE CHRISTIAN MARTYRS, YOU'VE COME!

TONITE'S THE NITE!

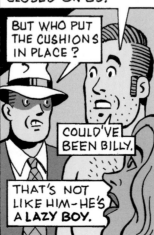

WE WERE COITUSSING SO HARD, THE SOFA BED CLOSED ON US.

BUT WHO PUT THE CUSHIONS IN PLACE?

COULD'VE BEEN BILLY.

THAT'S NOT LIKE HIM—HE'S A LAZY BOY.

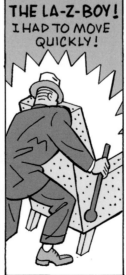

THE LA-Z-BOY! I HAD TO MOVE QUICKLY!

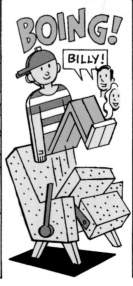

BOING!

BILLY!

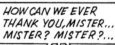

HOW CAN WE EVER THANK YOU, MISTER... MISTER? MISTER?...

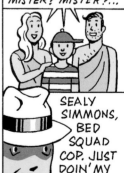

SEALY SIMMONS, BED SQUAD COP. JUST DOIN' MY JOB, FOLKS.

ASLEEP*

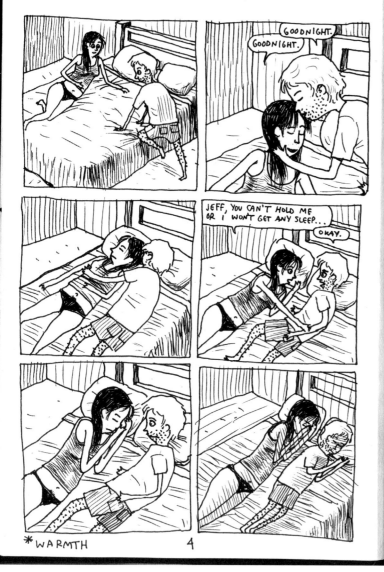

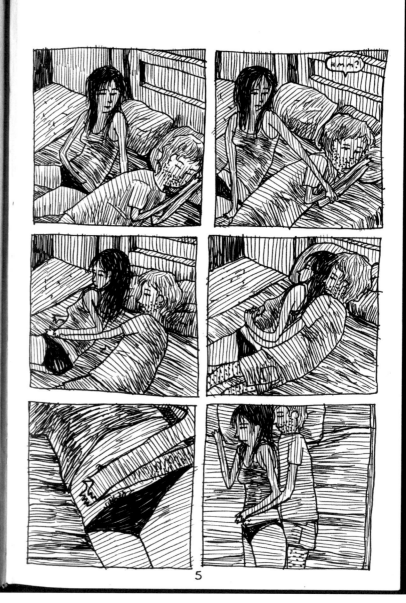

SOAK

BECKY MARGOLIS

Lucy wished she had taken something before they left, something to help her sleep and maybe a better book. There were no TVs where they were going, and Lucy had only brought the latest from her book club—the one that her sister urged her to join, and which she was now

regretting—a novel about conjoined vampire twins. She'd been stuck on page ten for the last week.

"It's so windy," Lucy said.

"That's just the sound of the car moving," Mitchell said. "It's not windy at all."

"It's really my least favorite type of weather. I wish it were snowing instead."

Mitchell kept his eyes on the road. "It doesn't snow in June," he said. "Not as long as I've lived here."

Lucy and Mitchell were going away for the weekend, but no, they were not going to get married. At some point, last week, or last

month, or last summer, Lucy had decided this. So, now what were they doing? They were taking a romantic trip, a few hours out of town, to Wild Horse Hot Springs Resort. It was a historic place, built in the 1940's and, according to their guidebook, featured 'leisurely vacations of the yesteryear.' They would spend the weekend *soaking*—like something dehydrated: beans or instant soup, water seeping in through their pores and the bottoms of their feet. Lucy imagined that they would emerge from the pool as versions of themselves fifty years from now, wrinkled and senile. Wrinkles so deep you could hoard raisins between them, or cherry pits.

Lucy pressed her face against the window, watching the empty rolling hills—like chubby, freckled knees—as they sped along the curvy two-lane highway, hugging the river. They passed the occasional car heading in the opposite direction and a few abandoned trucks littered along the side of the road. As they drove, the towns grew farther and farther apart and then seemed to disappear entirely. There were herds of cattle sprinkled sparingly across the landscape, dashed here as if on second thought, and even they looked spooked and disoriented.

"The mineral water in these pools can cure anything," Lucy said. "That's what I read on the website. Headaches, cancer—they have testimonials from customers."

"It's called advertising," Mitchell said.

Lucy didn't say anything more about the water after that, or the weather. These silences, when they first started cropping up in conversations not too long ago, used to bother Lucy, but lately she had begun to revel in them. She allowed the silence to fester, uninterrupted. It was a test of endurance, really—like trying to run to the next telephone pole before collapsing; holding your breath underwater until your lungs burst.

★ ★ ★

Who would you be, if you were in the story?

The one that's beautiful in an interesting sort of way: choppy haircut, misplaced freckles. Isn't she the one with the cat? Or is it a guinea pig?

Lucy can never remember the details right, which gets her into trouble. The other women—her sister's friends—accuse her of skimming, of pilfering these books for parakeets and broken furnaces and clever lines of dialogue. They suspect her of being a lazy reader. A book club thief. A sensationalist! They think she will go home and say to Mitchell: "Honey, I love you but when you touch me I crumble into a million pieces. Then you take the pieces, fry them in a pan, and eat me. Please don't eat me."

To be honest, Lucy would never steal something like that. Her sister and her friends are mistaken. The fact is, her life is already complicated enough as is. But the facts have a way of mixing themselves up. So to avoid any conflict, Lucy says, instead: I would be the last letter on every page.

★ ★ ★

They arrived finally at the town of Wild Horse. Signs along the highway declared its attractions: Healing waters! Live music! Espresso! The main strip featured a convenience store, a casino, a couple of restaurants and an out-of-business antiques shop. And on top of a small hill at the edge of town sat the resort, a faded pink, stucco building with two swimming pools in front, an empty field behind, and a bar next door, marked by a sign that read, *Get your beer here*. There were no horses to be seen, wild or otherwise. The place looked mostly deserted, just two or three

other cars besides theirs in the parking lot, and for a moment—with the wind howling wildly like that, and the thick gray sky, and the woman at the front desk who must have been a direct descendent of the wife from *The Shining*, it was the teeth really—Lucy wondered if they'd made some fatal mistake by coming here.

"Looks like you folks got here just before the weather," said the woman at the desk, as she handed them the room key. "Good timing."

"What's that smell?" Mitchell said. He raised his hand and swirled it around, as if to refer to the mild scent of rotten eggs hovering in the air.

"That's the bacteria in the water, converting to sulfur," the woman said.

Mitchell nodded, though he looked uncertain.

"The water in the pools here comes up from very deep inside the earth," she added.

"How deep?" Lucy said.

The woman smiled, showing off her large teeth, and said quietly, almost in a whisper, "As deep as a volcano."

Lucy didn't know what that meant. But she liked the sound of it. She pictured an underground river being pushed up through the dirt by bubbling lava—rivers on fire. "Does that make the water more potent?" she asked.

The woman shrugged. "Not sure," she said. "But people swear by it—have since the beginning of time." She paused and flicked her pencil against her palm. "You'll get used to the smell. Don't worry."

They walked back out to the car, grabbed their bags and went to find their room. Lucy opened the door and they stepped inside. "I don't want to wear my bikini out there," she said. "Everyone's going to look at me like I'm a whale."

Lucy had been growing, expanding from the waist out, right through her jeans and out of her dresses. She was filling herself with ice cream sandwiches and personal pan pizzas and Oreo cookies. A long time vegetarian, Lucy was now eating meat: burgers, hot dogs, bologna, whatever she could get. It had been a sudden transformation, just in the last six months or so, and Lucy believed she might have doubled in size, tripled even. But she was not scared. Lucy was intrigued by her rate of expansion, impressed even—like watching the way something molded if you left it out too long: where did that *stuff* come from?

"Maybe you're pregnant," her sister suggested.

"That's physically impossible," Lucy said.

One time, last year, Lucy had been pregnant for eight weeks, but her sister did not know this. During that time Lucy had felt as if there was some kind of magical sea urchin inside her, an urgent, dangerous secret. But when she learned that the baby had no heartbeat—when she lay on the examining chair watching the computer screen, the sonogram of the dead thing inside her—she'd been disgusted with her body. The failure of her organs, and the atrophied creature inside.

"You did the best you could," Mitchell had said, as if he were some sort of softball coach. "You didn't do anything wrong."

"No one's going to look at you," Mitchell said now, digging through his backpack, spilling its contents onto the bed like some mangled, useless thing. "Where the hell is my suit?"

"You can wear mine," Lucy said. "I'm not going in. I've got to finish reading, anyway."

"I could have sworn I packed it."

"You think no one looks at me anymore?"

"I can't believe I forgot my suit."

"Why do you keep calling it that—*suit*? What is it, a tux?"

"No," Mitchell said. "They're shorts."

Lucy sat down next to him on the bed. She ran her fingers over the rough, flowered comforter, tracing the seam. It was part of a mood, this comforter—maybe that's what a decorator would say—and the lace cloth on the night-stand, the dusty painting of a farm scene hanging above the vanity, the antique lamp. It all felt very forgotten, this room, this whole place, like they were here in the aftermath of a great party. The lingering presence of everyone who had slept in this bed: a king with tuberculosis, a duchess afflicted with rubella.

★ ★ ★

Were you sad when it was over? Did you feel like you were losing a friend?

Why sad? Couldn't you be relieved or satisfied or full or sick? Couldn't you be happy, even? Or does that mean there is something very wrong with you?

One woman, Charlene, is the one who clutches the book to her chest when she speaks. "I wish there was a sequel!"

Lucy pictures the ransom note they could compose: Give me another friend, or I'll never buy one of your books again. I'll slam you on my blog. You broke my heart.

The author would never write back. They'd move on to the next book: one with an unlikely hero, a boy who plucks out all his eyelashes and eyebrows. Lucy probably wouldn't finish it.

Sad? No, wouldn't use that word exactly. When it was over it felt, well, over. The ponies were a nice touch though, and the whole thing with the mother. Or was it the girlfriend? Hard to remember.

★ ★ ★

It would not be dark for a few hours still, and though Lucy felt anxious about exposing her thighs in the light of day, they decided to go for a short soak anyway. It was at least worth a shot: Lucy in her bikini and t-shirt, Mitchell in what used to be his jeans. Now the cut-offs ended mid-thigh.

"I think you cut these too short," Mitchell said.

"You look fine," Lucy said. Mitchell's legs were so white and skinny and hairy—like two lint-collecting wands at the very end of their life. "There's nobody else here anyway."

As it turned out, when they got down to the pools, unloaded their towels and water bottles on some nearby plastic lounge chairs, and removed their flip-flops, there were just a few other soakers. A middle-aged couple and their three kids, ranging in age from toddler to ten-year-old. They were all screaming about a juice-box, fighting over a foam noodle, peeing in the water. The father gave Lucy and Mitchell an apologetic smile and then a look that seemed to beg: can we switch places for a few hours?

Lucy considered it: the feeling of being in a man's body, of having a penis. The thought of having three small children, of being able to punch someone. It was not entirely unappealing. She looked over at Mitchell, standing awkwardly on the steps of the pool, water at ankle-level. He was squinting, like he was pretending to focus on something. The jeans were very short; the white pockets stuck out the bottom.

Mitchell and Lucy sat in the less hot pool of the two, which was more like lukewarm. There was a bench that lined the perimeter and Lucy imagined for a moment that every seat was occupied and the pool was full of soakers, the ghosts of the ailing. Lucy leaned her head back against the edge of the pool and looked up at the blanket of gray sky, which offered the promise of something terrible. She found this strangely comforting. For the first time in as long as she could remember, Lucy felt light—not weightless—but almost like there were strings attached to her limbs and the top of her head, and someone else, some giant puppeteer, was maneuvering them for her.

★ ★ ★

Five o'clock: more people began to arrive. A group of friends on a cross-country hot springs tour, some old men with liver-spotted shoulders, a young couple wearing bathing suits with matching tropical fish prints.

"I need to get out for a while," Mitchell said, holding up his arms, which were covered in small red bumps, a million tiny pimples. "Look, I've got a rash or something."

"It's all over your back too," Lucy said.

"There must be something in the water I'm allergic to," Mitchell said, climbing out of the pool. "Maybe it's the sulfur or something."

"I don't know," Lucy said. "I'm not a doctor."

Mitchell hoisted himself up onto the pool's ledge and sat there for a minute, dangling his legs into the water. "Do you want to come up to the room with me?" he said.

"I think I'll stay in a little longer," she said.

Mitchell frowned. "OK." He got completely out of the pool and grabbed his towel from the chair. "These jeans weigh about five pounds," he said.

Lucy watched Mitchell shuffle across the parking lot, towel wrapped over his shoulders

like a magician's cape. Sometimes Lucy wished that Mitchell would disappear, that he would simply cease to exist. And she knew that made her a terrible person, in a real sort of way.

"Looks like we've got a storm moving in," said one of the old men in the pool.

"Maybe," Lucy said.

"It's cold," he said. "I bet we'll see some snow."

Lucy shook her head. "Not what I've been told," she said. "It doesn't snow here in June."

★ ★ ★

Live music on the weekends: Lucy stood in the hotel lobby, listening to a young guy play the guitar. He was standing in the corner of the room and he sang into a microphone attached to a small amp. A poster on the wall explained that the musician was a local kid, from the town of Wild Horse itself.

"This one is for Colin," he said, and there was a somber applause from the audience—a crowd of maybe twenty people that had somehow slipped in while Lucy was out in the pool. Some were standing along the wall like she was; others sat on the hotel's antique couches that had been arranged in a semi-circle around the musician.

The kid began to play another sappy song. He was endearing though, Lucy had to admit. So small-town. He played the three chords, leaning his head to the side and closing his eyes. He sang

about Montana and the rivers and a woman. Who was Colin, Lucy wondered. Colin. Colin. She said the name a few times in her head, letting her tongue touch the roof of her mouth as she did. Lucy liked the sound of it; she'd like to give a turtle that name, or a cactus, maybe.

When the song was over, Lucy walked across the room, past the front desk and toward the stairs. She should check on Mitchell—make sure that he was still breathing, that his entire body wasn't swollen or eating itself. But before heading up, she walked back through the lobby and outside, where she grabbed her phone and the cigarette that was stashed in the pocket of her sweatshirt. She lit it, taking a couple deep drags before dialing.

"Well hello, Lucy," he said, picking up after four rings. "How the hell are you?"

It was an old friend, Greg—an old boyfriend, really—who she spoke to a few times a year, sometimes more, depending on how lonely or bored she was feeling.

"Oh," Lucy said. "I'm great."

"Glad to hear it."

"I masturbated to you last night," she said, which wasn't true.

Greg let out a couple short, hard laughs. She'd made him uncomfortable. "You did?"

"Is that funny to you?"

"No, no. I mean, it just surprised me."

"I see," Lucy said. "The thing is, I've gotten huge now."

"Huge?"

"Yes, like imagine there are two of me on one pair of legs."

"Hmm, that's hot."

"Not exactly."

"Hey—let me get *my* masturbation material."

Lucy glanced around the parking lot, suddenly worried that someone might be eavesdropping. She put out her cigarette. "I'm visiting some hot springs," she said.

"Why are you whispering?"

"Sorry," Lucy said, raising her voice. "Do you know anything about hot springs?"

"Who are you there with—Mitchell?"

"They basically start as volcanoes underground. Isn't that fascinating?"

"Yeah, sure," Greg said. "Listen Lucy, not to be an asshole, but what are you sticking around for?"

"We're having a good time."

"Haven't you been talking about leaving this guy for months now?"

Lucy sighed. It was true, most of her conversations with Greg did revolve around her inability to leave Mitchell. And Greg listened, he offered advice—likely yielded from his own experiences—from when he'd left her. "It's complicated," she said.

"You don't have to settle, Lucy. You deserve to be happy."

"Yeah well, thanks."

"Come to Chicago. I'll take care of you."

His offer—and he always offered—was somewhat appealing. Being taken care of sounded nice. He made it seem simple, obvious even.

"I couldn't move to Chicago," Lucy said. "I hate the wind."

"Well, if things change, you've got my number," Greg said. "It's a beautiful city, I'm telling you. And great baseball."

★ ★ ★

Mitchell was alive, though not well. Lucy found him passed out on his stomach across the bed, still in his jean shorts—still wet.

"Why don't you take these off?" Lucy said, nudging him.

Mitchell grumbled and rolled over. "Where were you?"

"I was listening to music. There's a kid playing guitar downstairs."

"You smell like cigarettes."

"Sorry," she said. Her heart jumped, and for a second she felt like she was in trouble. "How's your rash?"

Mitchell held up his arms, which were still covered in red bumps. It looked worse than before. There were so many bumps Lucy could not even count them if she tried.

"Should we go to the hospital?" Lucy said.

"No, no," Mitchell said. "I just need to sleep. That smell is making me sick."

"What smell?"

"The fart smell," Mitchell said. "The rotten eggs."

"I don't even notice it anymore."

"I have a heightened sense of smell," Mitchell said. "You know this."

In fact, she did—Mitchell was like one of those cop dogs: first to notice when there was wet laundry mildewing in the washing machine, when the cookies were burning, or when a shower was overdue. It was oddly comforting, this consistency—to know that she wouldn't ever have to worry about burnt baked goods, about eating the entire batch alone—wasn't it?

"I'm bored," Lucy said. She stood up from the bed. "I don't understand; we're just supposed to sit in these hot pools all evening. What are we waiting around for?"

"Hey, be happy you don't have a rash."

"I'm not happy," she said. "I don't think the water here is going to fix anything."

Mitchell scratched his arms with determination. The skin became much redder, shiny almost. His fingernails were very short, like a dull cheese grater.

Lucy winced. "Stop scratching, please."

"Sorry." Mitchell dropped his hands on the bed.

They sat there silently for a while then. The silence grew—expanded to fill the whole room, all the way to the door and into Lucy's stomach. She glanced down at her hands and noticed that her fingers looked like sausages. She wanted to bite them, see how difficult it might be to chew them off.

"Go back to the pool if you want," Mitchell said, rolling over onto his back. He stared up at the ceiling, arms at his sides like a corpse.

"What are we waiting for?" Lucy said, again.

Mitchell shrugged. "It's not like you wake up one day and something happens," he said. "You don't even realize something's happened until after it does."

★ ★ ★

Does this remind you of a dream you've had?

Always, it does; or a movie, or a fantasy, or a past life in India. Everyone wants to relate—to share their story about the story. Charlene knows a friend who has a sister that lived in the same town as the main character. Lucy's sister once had an out-of-body experience—after sitting in a sauna for too long—in which she envisioned this same story, *exactly*, except backwards. She calls it karma.

Once, a long time ago, Lucy had a dream about becoming a blimp—of inflating to huge proportion and floating above all the highest skyscrapers, above the clouds and airplanes like a huge balloon. It was peaceful and frightening at the same time. It was like swimming, like almost drowning. She had tried to recall this feeling the next morning, but couldn't.

★ ★ ★

Both pools began to empty out again, people going home, to bed. It was dark, but Lucy couldn't see the stars. On the other side of the pool sat the kid who had been playing guitar earlier in the hotel lobby. The local celebrity. He looked different with his hair wet though, without the microphone—younger, maybe. And because he felt familiar to Lucy somehow, or maybe just because she was curious, she scooted around the bench until she was sitting next to him. He looked over and raised his eyebrows in greeting.

"Hi," Lucy said. "I heard you play earlier. It was good. I liked it."

"Thanks," he said. He stared out across the pool and then back at Lucy. His eyes were big and dark and he didn't seem to blink.

Lucy slid her toes back and forth a few times across the concrete bottom. It felt like sandpaper rubbing against the soles of her feet, in a good way. A couple of bright spotlights hung from tall posts around the pool area and shined down on all of them, illuminating the surface of the water and the tops of their wet heads with streaks of fluorescence.

Lucy looked back at the musician. A piece of hair hung down in his face and she resisted the urge to brush it away, to tuck it carefully behind his ear. "I was wondering," she said, "Who is Colin—who you played that song for? A cactus?"

The kid laughed. "What?"

"It sounds like a good cactus name."

He shook his head. "No, Colin was a friend of mine," he said. Then he paused. "He died last month though."

"Oh jeez," Lucy said. "Sorry about that. I mean, sorry for calling him a cactus, too."

"That's alright."

"How did he die?"

The guitar player looked surprised, at first. Then he ran his tongue along his teeth. "He walked off a cliff," he said. "In his sleep."

"Really?" Lucy said. It sounded like a myth, a story. Like something she might read in a book, something to which her sister might declare: not possible, not in real life. "Is that true?"

"Colin was backpacking in South Dakota, camping near the edge of a tall overhang." The guitar player lifted up his skinny arms and rested his elbows on the edge of the pool, dangling his fingers into the water.

"Wait," Lucy said. "How do you know he didn't do it on purpose?" But after the words left her mouth, she felt like punching herself. "Sorry, that was inappropriate."

"Colin was a sleepwalker. A sleep-*runner*, actually. One time he ran three miles to the store in his sleep, bought a pack of gum, and ran home. He wasn't the kind of person that was depressed."

Lucy shivered, even though it wasn't cold, and skimmed her hand along the surface of the water, watching the little rivers that peeled off her fingers. "This water came from a volcano," she said.

He took a sip of something in a water bottle.

"What's that?" she said.

"Water."

"Do you think he woke up?" Lucy said. "While he was falling, I mean. Do you think he was awake when he hit the ground?"

The guitar player—Colin's friend, whose name Lucy did not even know—didn't say anything at first. "I think so," he finally said. "He must have woken up. When I'm falling in my dreams, I always wake up before I hit the ground."

"You're right," Lucy said. "That's the most terrifying thing I can imagine."

As homage to this, or something like it, Lucy dunked her head under the water. It felt like little knives on her eyelids. She tried to hold her head there as long as she could, but when the sharp pressure started to subside, she ran out of breath. She lifted her head up quickly and wiped her eyes, gasping.

The kid stared at Lucy, like he thought that she was a crazy woman. Maybe she was; maybe the sulfur was getting to her, too. She checked her arms for rashes—for evidence of something affected—but they looked fine.

"Look," said the guitar player. He was pointing out into the dark—or rather, to the beam under the spotlight, where they could see a flurry of snowflakes: chunky, unrelenting, falling in metered rows. And then, to the quietly disrupted surface of the pool, where the flakes paused momentarily before dissolving into the water.

★ ★ ★

What is this really about?

The first question every week, to get things going. As if the story is about something *else*, as if things are happening somewhere that aren't really happening. Cars are crashing into each other, but no one is dying. Leaves are falling, but there aren't any piles. People are licking popsicles, but they don't have tongues.

Lucy sometimes imagines a ticker tape running below every minute of her life, detailing each step and misstep, like subtitles. But that's the kind of thing that will drive a person crazy, in the real sense of the word. Squashing a bug with a penny, making strong coffee, then hearing a song on the neighbor's radio: what's all that *really* about?

What it's really about is giving voice to the tongue-less.

So Lucy wants to know: could you speak at all, without a tongue? Could you scream?

"Just shout it out," says Lucy's sister. "There aren't any right answers here."

Lucy thinks this might be good advice, generally. Like in crowded elevators, the middle of empty gymnasiums, or into someone's ear when they are sleeping. It takes some of the pressure off, doesn't it—knowing that you can't be right?

And then, like popcorn: lovelovelovelovelovelovelove!

Lucy opened the door to the hotel room. It was dark, but the blinds were open and the

lights outside by the pools and the parking lot illuminated the room with a murky glow. Mitchell was a lump under the covers, snoring lightly.

She took off her shoes and her wet bathing suit, shivering, and felt around in the dark for her bag—for some dry clothes. She put on her sweater and a pair of socks.

Tomorrow, they would drive home. There would be several inches of snow on the roads, but it would all melt by noon—any evidence of the strange, of the illicit cold, would be gone before they even left. In fact, it would be sunny, and they would drive with the windows down, with the music turned up. Past the hills and the cows and the volcanoes underground. Lucy would leave her book in the hotel—perhaps accidentally—on the little table next to the bed. She would wait to see what happened.

WHAT THEY'RE SAYING

ROBERT DUFFER

They're saying he lit himself on fire while his wife lay in bed. Firefighters found a gas can in the master bedroom, where the mother died of smoke inhalation, as did the middle child, a son, in the adjacent room. The suicide note, set neatly beside his will on the garage floor, said it all:

he was sorry and he wanted to take the whole family with him.

But the eldest, a daughter of twelve, leapt from an upstairs window to get help for her youngest brother, six, who waited on the roof as smoke billowed out of the windows. The father was found in the kitchen, with a gash in his head and burns covering 100% of his body[1]; he would die the next day.

It's the kind of story met with disbelief. Not just the tragedy itself but in the unsettled wake of the tragedy, when we feel the shades of doubt being pulled down on even the most intimate relationships. What happens behind the closed doors of our neighbors—these strangers we presume to know through shared circumstance, this tenuous fiber of community—is not something we know. To know it is to open that door of possibility in ourselves: how precarious is the difference between who we are, the image we project, and who we could be, the shadows we cage?

The mother was a guidance counselor at area high schools. The father, an artist known for his landscapes, worked from home. The gallery owner who hosted the artist's shows said the father belied no trace of depression, as authorities asserted, when asking about

his sales[2]. Credible quotes were mined from friends, coworkers, their preacher from the local Catholic church—where they were active if not devout—all saying dumbstruck that he was a loving father, coached his son's teams, there was nothing wrong, no marital problems. But really, what trusted friend, with access to the intimacies of their relationship, would tell the media about their problems on the night of their death?

The story the community is telling is horrific and haunting, yes, but most of all it is understandable. Struggling artist with a history of depression finally snaps under economic hard times. An artist, eccentric, enigmatic, a flake. Afflicted with a mental disease, unstable, unpredictable, unsafe. The storyline plays to our prejudices, the skepticism of an artist making a living and sustaining a family. We choose what we want to believe. It explains the inexplicable, answers the unanswerable why.

But the narrative feels flawed. Why would a self-employed artist cite financial difficulties as the reason to murder his family when he'd been able to sustain his art and his family for nearly 15 years in a middle-income suburb? Wouldn't most artists envy that level of success? To be fair, how much of my skepticism stems from being a stay-at-home parent and artist, like the alleged immolator?

Curious events in the garage. Firefighters arrived at 3:30am. An hour earlier, the wife made a call from her cell phone; she rammed her minivan into the garage door, then left it askew in the garage. The garage, where the gas can would be, where the suicide note was. She goes back inside. To protect the children from the madman that coached their teams, led church retreats and was inspired by French landscapists? Why did she go back? Was she enraged or was she scared?

Would she know why she went back?

The eldest, the daughter, said she was getting out of bed to get a glass of water when she heard a 'pop' and the hallway filled with smoke. Then she jumped out of the second story window.

The daughter's glass-of-water story is a likely one from a tween who doesn't want everyone to know how her parents fight. Her brother, rescued by the neighbor from the roof, said he heard their mom vomiting as they escaped from the window. The smoke was thick. Mom was up, hacking, crying, vomiting[3]? But ultimately still in bed, doing nothing.

"Fires don't 'pop,'" my friend the fireman said. Firemen don't talk about their jobs to non-firemen. They're reticent unless drunk. And he was, on the fish-tail end of a pub crawl. I asked about the head trauma. He raised his eyebrows yes, indicating there was more. He wasn't even there, yet all the firemen are saying the same thing, "You just know" when it doesn't add up, he said.

Let's say this time, the fighting ends abruptly, ends with a pop. A pop not like a fire but a pop like a head being hit. Maybe, ablaze, he hit his

head on the counter. Or maybe he got hit by a golf club or a baseball bat or another blunt object from the garage. Maybe the mom had something to hide he was about to expose.

Why, if he wanted to take everyone with him, did he light himself on fire then stumble down the hall, down the stairs to the nearest exit? If it's difficult to know the inner thoughts of a man, then let's agree it's impossible to know the thoughts of a man on fire.

The suicide note mutes all suspicion. That was the lynchpin, laid out neatly beside his will in the garage. At least one source claimed that he had attempted suicide before[4]; had he left a note then? Could the note have been an emotional response to an adulterous wife? Could it have been contrived by the wife?

Could be. Or the prevailing version of the truth, that the father did it, is in fact what happened. It's much easier to believe, much better to insulate ourselves from the ultimate unknowing and for the community to say it was the depressive artist and not the mother counseling the youth at our high schools who tried to burn his family.

We don't know; you never do. We'll agree on a narrative and stop talking about it because it isn't our story. It belongs to the kids that survived; it's theirs forever.

1. http://dailyherald.com/story/?id=297826
2. http://www.chicagobreakingnews.com/2009/06/arlington-heights-fire-kills-woman-boy.html
3. http://articles.chicagotribune.com/2009-06-04/news/0906030958_1_pinewood-derby-garrett-suicide-note
4. http://articles.chicagotribune.com/2009-06-04/news/0906030958_1_pinewood-derby-garrett-suicide-note

THE SLEEPWALKER

THE RESIDENTS

People say you can only see ghosts through the corner of your eye, but it's not true. I've seen the ghost of my wife right in front of me—the first time was not too long after I killed her.

I guess I should explain. I'm a sleepwalker, and apparently, I'm a violent sleepwalker. Yes, as I said at the trial, we weren't getting along so well when it happened, but I loved Maggie and I'd never do anything to harm her—well, I guess that's not true. I killed her, after all.

Maggie told me that I walked in my sleep, but I didn't believe her. She loved to find things to pick at me about—she did it all the time—pick, pick, pick. Your bald spot is getting bigger, don't leave your dirty clothes on the bedroom floor, those pants make you look fat. After a while you just get used to it—and you don't hear it anymore. Then, of course, she finds something

worse, and that's what I figured was happening with sleepwalking—it was just something new to pick on me about. Until she put the flour on the floor.

See, the idea was that putting flour on the floor was the ultimate test. If we woke up the next morning and there were footprints in the flour and the soles of my feet were white, then that would be it—absolute proof. So we did and they were—white, that is. I hated it. Maggie was so fucking arrogant, what could I say? So I refused to believe it. I mean her feet were almost as big as mine. She could have made those footprints, then cleaned herself up and

smeared some flour on my feet. I'm a pretty heavy sleeper, after all. I wouldn't have put it past her.

So I came up with another test. This time she would sleep on the couch and I would lock the bedroom door before dusting the floor with flour. That way, the next morning, if there were footprints and flour on my feet, sleepwalking would be the only explanation. I woke up early the next day feeling oddly refreshed and excited, until I looked down and saw the footprints on the floor, along with my undeniably white feet. Dejected, I then unlocked the bedroom door, and followed my footprints from the kitchen into the living room, where I found Maggie lying on the carpet, a bloody butcher knife next to her twisted and lifeless body. I don't know how I did it without waking little Becky, our daughter, but there didn't seem to be any doubt about what happened. I mean, I pretty much proved it myself.

But I got a smart lawyer, and he got me off. I guess I got away with murder, or at least that's what everyone said. But the thing is, I don't remember any of it. Yeah, I guess I did it and I feel really bad about what happened, but it wasn't like I planned it all out or anything.

But then her ghost started showing up. The first time, I had to get up in the middle of the night to take a piss and there she was in the hall, just staring at me with this kind of slightly evil, slightly self-righteous grin. She was just like you always see in the movies—kind of whitish and slightly transparent—and then she disappeared. POOF! Just like that, she was gone. Well, I figured it was a dream or something and forgot about it.

But then...but then, a couple of weeks later, I woke up again and there was little Becky, standing at the foot of my bed—sleepwalking, with her eyes wide open. It was spooky as hell. I picked her up and put her back in her room, but then it happened again. This time, I heard her talking, talking to Maggie. They were in the kitchen, talking about knives. Maggie told her which ones are the sharpest and showed her how to hold a knife, and then when she started telling her about the eyes, arteries, and vital organs—exactly where to cut and stab—I ran into the room. Of course, Maggie's ghost vanished and left little Becky standing there, that spooky blank look on her face and a knife in her hand. When I asked her about it the next day, she couldn't remember a thing.

And now I guess it's just a matter of time. Three of my sharpest knives are missing; I've searched the whole house, but I can't find them anywhere. Every night, when I go to sleep, I lock the bedroom door, but sooner or later I'll sleepwalk again and she'll be out there, waiting for me.

A THIRD OF YOUR LIFE

MEGAN STIELSTRA

People throw the word crazy around a lot—*those kids are crazy! What are you, crazy? I'm going crazy!*—but I know what crazy really means because of this guy Tom. He lives above the breakfast place where I work, and every day he comes downstairs to eat. He's a big dude:

shaved head, moustache, and he only wears cutoff jean shorts and knee-high suede moccasins with fringe. That's all, so you can *really* see his whole nine yards: hairy back, flabby front, he sweats a lot—Appetizing? Not so much. My boss, Josh, gave him the whole *no shoes no shirt no service* song and dance so Tom went out and got a suede fringed vest that matched the moccasins. I figure he must freeze in the winter and now, one of those awful Chicago Julys, he's *got* to be dying under all that animal skin—but it isn't my place to ask. What I can ask is, "You want some coffee, Tom?"

"Absolutely not," he always says. "I don't condone that sort of behavior." Then

he goes on to explain what caffeine can do if you mix it with other chemicals—Lithium or Prozac or Wellbutrin or Lexapro or Celexa specifically, 'cause those are the ones he's on.

"Okay, then," I say, and get him juice instead. Then a red pepper benedict, the Garden section of the *Trib*, and two crossword puzzles. After that he gets up, lays down a twenty, and goes to work at the Sealy Posturepedic warehouse, driving pillows around in a great big truck.

"How's your mattress, Megan?" he asks me, very seriously.

"It's fine," I say, 'cause what else do you say?

"Gotta be," he says. "You spend a third of your life on your mattress."

I don't know if he realizes that we've had this same conversation, right down to the sentence structure, for nearly a year; that because of him I can define such terms as *Depressive Pseudodementia* and *Psychomotor Retardation* with medical exactitude. It's actually helpful, this front row seat to crazy, 'cause lately I've been thinking I might be going crazy myself.

★ ★ ★

Every morning, I get to the restaurant at six a.m. I walk from table to table, putting napkins down at every right corner. Then I take the same walk, putting spoons on the right side of every napkin. Then, around again with knives, and then—*then*—the forks. *Napkin spoon knife fork napkin spoon knife fork* and I've been working here for, what, five years now? I never was very good at math, but that's a lot of forks, right? *Right?* So what would happen if I switched it up a bit? Maybe go napkin *fork* knife spoon, or knife *then* fork, or maybe really let loose and put the forks on the *right* side of the napkin—Would the world start spinning backwards? Would the glaciers melt or meteors crash or humanity find some common ground— who knows? *Not me!* So last week, on Monday, I put down all forks. No knives or spoons, just three forks on every napkin. Then, on Tuesday, I didn't put down any forks at all, just all knives and

spoons, and on Wednesday, no spoons. So maybe you're thinking *This isn't very interesting, Megan, I've got better things to think about than cutlery*—and I get it, I do—but it's important that you stick with me here 'cause this is how I lost my mind. For real. Not *Oh I'm going crazy* like we say eight hundred times a day, but serious. *Certifiable*.

"Uhm, Megan?" Molly asked after a few days of resetting the silverware I'd just set. She'd never dream of second-guessing me—she's only been working here a couple months and I've been here five years—Five years, waiting tables at the same exact place—*five*. "What are you doing?"

"I don't know, Molly," I said. I turned around and faced her, her curly hair and careful smile and fistfuls of forks. "Maybe I'm going crazy."

She laughed. "Totally," she said. "That happens to me all the time."

I pointed a fork at her and said, "I'm serious, Molly. I might be seriously crazy."

★ ★ ★

"You're seriously crazy," Andy said, when I suggested we go dancing. We'd just picked up some take-out from Penny's Noodles and were driving back to his place.

"Let's go!" I said again, having that fun little fantasy where you've got a rose between your teeth and your boyfriend's in tight black pants with a magical wonderful ass, dipping you low and dragging you slowly up his torso. "I saw a sign back there, let's try it!"

He stopped at a red light and turned to face me. "I'm from Marquette Park," he said, as if the South Side was where this question would die. "Besides," he went on. "It's almost time for CSI."

This is what we do, me and Andy. We get take-out food and go home at the end of a long day, mine at the restaurant and his the ad firm. We snuggle up on the couch and drink beers and relax. He'll have one arm around me, and sometimes we'll make out, and if that gets heavy we'll go into the bedroom for sex, after which he falls asleep fast 'cause he works all these hours, and that's when I lay there, listening to him breathe. It's something between breathing and snoring, actually, with a little bit of spit rolling in the back of his throat. Sometimes he whistles through his nose. I listen to this every night.

Every night.

Every night.

Every night and then the alarm goes off at five and I'm at work by six, setting up the restaurant: *napkin spoon knife fork*, creamers in the bowls, "What kind of toast would you like with that, sir?" and in my hands are the coffee cups. I imagine throwing them, or flinging plates like Frisbees, they'd smash against the wall right above the line of customers' heads and it would be so, so, so satisfying but instead I say, "Would you like hash browns or side salad?" to the three-top at table seven and "Citrus vinaigrette or lemon tarragon?" to the lady on nineteen and to Tom I say, "You want some coffee?"

"I don't condone such behavior," he says, and

this is our routine. Pepper benedicts, crossword puzzles, *a third of your life on a mattress* and on we go, every day, Monday through Friday. Tom never comes in on the weekends. On the weekends, it's not breakfast but *brunch*. Brunch in Chicago is an almost religious experience. The restaurant is packed, people wait over an hour for a table—it's way too much for Tom to handle.

★ ★ ★

The day it happened was a Sunday, one of those awful 90-degree mornings where the humidity wraps over you like a blanket. All the customers waited inside for their tables, to be near the a/c, and me and Molly and the other girls could barely shove through the bodies. "Excuse me!" we said, carrying plates high over our heads. "Coming though! Look out, this stains!" I was behind the counter pouring mimosas when Tom came in, all bare hairy chest and dangly fringe. He looked shocked to see so many people, here, in *his* place, *his* breakfast, *his* routine. I saw him talk to Josh by the front door. I couldn't hear them over all the people, but I figured Josh told him he'd have to wait.

That wouldn't go over very well.

Tom stood for a minute, oblivious to the stares he was getting 'cause of his clothes, and then turned to the nearest customer—some dad with a comb-over and pleated pants. *Don't,* I thought, not knowing what he was doing but sure that he shouldn't as he grabbed the guy's arm and

whispered something. The dad's eyes widened, and he backed up a couple steps into the lady behind him. A sort of domino effect happened then—customers backing into busboys backing into waitresses with Tom moving forward through the mayhem, grabbing anyone who got in his way, whispering something to each of them, and eventually he made it to the counter—to me. His eyes were glazed, a thin layer of milk coating the iris, and I knew he wasn't seeing me as he wrapped one meaty fist around my elbow and tightened, his fingers pushing through my skin, hitting bone and it hurt, it hurt, but I knew he wouldn't hear me if I said, "Let me go, Tom," or "You want some coffee, Tom?" or "Did you forget the Lexapro this morning, Tom?" He wouldn't hear my words 'cause he didn't hear his own, like somebody else was speaking through his mouth as he whispered, "If you don't get out of here, I'll take you outside and smash your head on the sidewalk. I'll hold it between my palms and pound it into the concrete."

When I think back on this, I don't remember feeling scared. I remember feeling sad. He was so completely alone.

★ ★ ★

In the end, Josh called the cops and Tom was 86ed—couldn't come into the restaurant without an automatic arrest. I'd see him sometimes, driving the big 'ol Sealy truck packed with pillows, and he'd always ask how my mattress was.

"Gotta be fine," he'd say. "You spend a third of your life on a mattress," and I'd repeat those words at night—a *third of your life, a third of your life*—as I listened to Andy breathe, the spit-sloggy in and outs, feeling my mattress below me, watching the ceiling above me, watching the clock: one o'clock, two o'clock, three, and by then I was imagining all the things I could stick up Andy's nose: drinking straws, uncapped Sharpies, the corkscrew for wine—and one night, a month or so after Tom went crazy, I got out of bed and went to the kitchen. I opened the silverware drawer and took out the knives and forks and spoons, and then I opened the oven and stuck them all in. There was still a lot of space in there, so I got the dishes and put them in, too, and the pots and pans, and the blender and the electric juicer and everything on the spice rack, and by then there was too much stuff in the oven, so I took it all out and tried to put it back in a rational manner, like when you're packing for some big trip. You roll up the underwear and the socks and stuff them in your running shoes. You put the extra batteries in with your toiletries. You fold your flip-flops into your sweaters—you make it fit. I would make it fit. *Fit,* goddammit! And suddenly, the overhead light came on and there was Andy standing over me.

I've since tried to imagine what he saw that night—the girl he thought he knew so well, squatting on the tiled kitchen floor with her blue nightgown hiked up around her thighs, surrounded by foodstuffs and spices and flatware

and Tupperware. My eyes must have been glassy as I looked up at him, my hair wild.

He was very still as he sized me up. Then he asked, "What's going on in here?" as though I might have a logical explanation.

"Your nose whistles," I said.

He just stood there, not making any sudden movements.

"—Every night," I went on. "Every night it whistles, every night I listen, and I figured I should get up this time and do something different so that every night wouldn't be the same night as last night—"

That's when the alarm starts buzzing in our bedroom, and it's time to go to work. *Napkin spoon fork knife.* Creamers in the bowls. Coffee decaf regular and at nine-thirty we open and the place fills up. It doesn't matter where my mind is—my body knows what to do. It's muscle memory that makes your latte, classical conditioning that reaches for the juice, like how someone can ask, *What's up?* and you say, *Fine,* 'cause you assume they've said, *How are you?*

I know what to do and I do it—it's routine—except today is different. Today Molly says,

"Hey, look," and points out the front windows of the restaurant. It's one of those warm perfect Chicago September mornings—every customer waiting for a table is standing around *outside*: moms and dads, girlfriends and boyfriends, tables of six or seven friends meeting for brunch, all of them on the sidewalk looking at the sky with their arms in the air and their hands held palms up to catch the snow. Snow—it's snowing—white fluffy flakes falling mid-September—but when I get closer to the windows and out the front door, I can see what it really is—feathers. Hundreds of feathers floating in the air, and I stand on the sidewalk and tilt my head back. There, leaning out his window above us with an army knife and a pillow, is Tom in all his fringe. He splits the pillow open with the knife, holds two opposite corners and shakes it 'til the feathers fly. Then he reaches behind him and grabs another pillow, pillow after pillow. "How's your mattress, Megan?" he yells down from the window, and I close my eyes and let the feathers brush my face.

It feels really wonderful.

Even if it is kind of crazy.

INTERVIEW: JOE LO TRUGLIO

WHAT HAVE YOU LOST THE MOST SLEEP OVER IN YOUR LIFE?

Joe Lo Truglio: Most recently it's been do I take Jamaal Charles or LeSean McCoy with the 4th overall pick in my fantasy draft. But in terms of things that matter, things that truly warrant deep retrospection, it usually revolves around whether or not I'm "doing enough." This covers everything: work, relationships, my health, general "fellow man" contributions. It's hard for me to rest. I can relax, but it's hard for me to rest. Effortlessness breeds suspicion in me. Which is silly, of course, but I'm wired that way. I love naps for this reason. In the day, it's easier for me to accept sleep as just another appointment. A by-product of productivity. It becomes a pause button, rather than a reset. Enjoying the reset is the thing to learn. "Enjoying The Reset" is also a wonderfully banal title for a self-help book.

ANY FOND (OR FUNNY OR AWKWARD OR ANYTHING REALLY) MEMORIES/ANECDOTES OF SHOOTING A SCENE IN A BED?

Joe Lo Truglio: When I was a kid, I made a movie called *Mexican Chainsaw Massacre* and I coerced my dad to be in it. At the end of the movie, the killer's dad—my father—wakes his son and says, "Now it is *your* turn, my son..!" and chainsaws him in the bed. My buddy Bobby, who played the killer, and I couldn't stop laughing. Between my dad's line reading

and the fact that it was ridiculous that a guy with a loud, roaring chainsaw can "sneak up" on his sleeping victim was just too much.

DO YOU HAVE ANY RECURRING DREAMS OR THEMES THAT POP UP REGULARLY?

Joe Lo Truglio: I used to have dreams as a kid of being swept off my feet from behind and violently pushed toward the moon. The moon would have this mean, judgmental "old man" face. It was terrifying. I often dream about subways, underground corridors. About twice a year, I'll dream about my teeth either falling out or floating out of my mouth.

WHERE'S THE STRANGEST PLACE YOU'VE EVER SLEPT?

Joe Lo Truglio: Me and a few from the guys from *The State* went to Greece back in 1995. In Athens we had about two or three hours to kill with nowhere to stay and we were pretty beat from the night before. We took a nap in a seedy, derelict-filled park with our knapsacks lying about. It was also about 103 degrees. Thinking about it now, it wasn't so much "strange"' as it was, "the stupidest fucking move ever."

SOCK ADDICTION

BRANDI WELLS

My friend Joe has been sneaking into department stores so he can cum in all the socks. "You're never going to cum in them all," I tell him, but he's convinced he can. He carries dirty magazines with him and sometimes watches videos on his iPhone and eventually

convinces me to go with him.

We stand between aisles and he pulls a few white athletic socks off the rack. He unclips them and unzips his pants. I turn and look at the rack of socks, peeking through to see if there's anyone nearby.

"Hike up your skirt a little," he tells me.

I don't and he repeats his request, but louder.

I'm afraid someone will come over and see him jacking off into a sock, so I pull my skirt up a little.

"A little more," he says and I do. Soon my skirt's around my waist and he's asking about my underwear.

★ ★ ★

We make the rounds twice a week and rotate stores, so it doesn't look suspicious. And I start wearing tights, so pulling up my skirt won't be so revealing, but he convinces me to take them off too. So I stand in the sock section, tights dangling in my hand, while he's smack, smack, smack. I worry someone will hear him, so sometimes I pretend we're having a conversation.

"We should probably try to grab lunch early," I say.

"Maybe we can see a movie," I add.

He tells me to be quiet. Not in a mean way, but maybe the way a mother tells their kid to be quiet when she's trying to watch television or read a book. Or trying to get off.

★ ★ ★

Joe used to have a porn addiction. He kept it on loop in his room and had to take breaks in stores and restaurants the way chain smokers do, so he could watch a little porn and try to get off. But lately he hasn't been watching it. It's just the socks in the department stores. I feel like it's an improvement. I mean, only twice a week isn't that bad. And we can finish our meals and movies without his constant need for a break.

★ ★ ★

My mother asks me if Joe and I are dating and I'm not sure what to say.

"I mean, what's dating?" I ask.

"Dinner," she says. "Movies. He pays. You hold hands."

"Maybe we're dating," I say.

She asks me to invite him for dinner and I say maybe to that too. It seems possible now since he can make it through dinners without the constant breaks.

★ ★ ★

I start dressing up for our trips to the department stores. I buy lace underwear, thongs at first

and then the crotch-less sort. I work out so my thighs will be toned and my ass will be firm. He appreciates it. I can tell because he fills almost twice as many socks. He holds my hand afterwards and I help him return the socks to their display rack.

We've gotten the timing down, so I don't worry so much about people catching us anymore. We know when the clerks' breaks are and when they're busy at the front. I still worry about another customer stumbling upon us, but most people are willing to give us the benefit of the doubt. They want to believe they didn't see what they saw. So they keep quiet and leave us alone.

But after a few months Joe seems less interested. He doesn't ask me to hike up my skirt and when I do anyway, he doesn't look. He just jacks off into the socks. He doesn't say a word. I help him put the socks up and he holds my hand loosely for a few seconds before he lets it go. And after a few more weeks, he quits calling me to go with him. I follow him and stand an aisle over and peek at him through the racks. He jacks off into a sock while rubbing another across his chest. I think he sees me, but he doesn't say anything and we don't make eye contact.

Part of me wants to go get a sales clerk. I want to tell them what he's been doing. Point at him. Show them how dirty and wrong he is. They'll make him stop. They'll put up signs with his picture on it. If he tries to come into the store, a guard will drag him outside and throw him into

the street. But I don't. I leave as he starts what looks like round two.

★ ★ ★

I drive over to Joe's house to wait on him, so we can talk. He never talks anymore. A survey of his room reveals home videos of socks. Bags of socks I didn't know he had. Socks arranged in suggestive positions. A sock with a pink ribbon tied around it. I throw the socks away and I leave.

I check his room again after a few days and he has new socks. More socks than before. Dark socks and white socks. Boys' socks. Girls' socks. Socks with toes. And videos of socks are running on loop on his laptop. His mp3 player is turned down low, but it's playing Marvin Gaye.

LIKE HOLDING A LITTLE BIRD

LAURYN ALLISON LEWIS

Her bedroom is no bigger than a small walk-in closet. She sleeps on a twin-sized mattress on the floor, around which there are no more than six inches of floor space in any direction. She hangs her clothes on a hot water pipe that bisects the room. The building she lives in is

very old; doors do not fit cozily in their jambs. Often during the night we are awoken by the sounds of a door creaking open of its own volition, the effect is ghostly.

She lives with four men, all of whom look hungry about the eyes, skin gray and tight, mossy teeth, greasy hair. She tells me to ignore them, and I try. Most nights they sit around on milk crates which double as living room furniture and storage for their copious collections of obscure records. They are in noize bands or math rock bands. They are performance artists. In other words, they are unemployed. Their girlfriends have not-so-secret heroin addictions. Their girlfriends are makeup artists, or freelance models who never smile during photo shoots.

We spend as much time as possible at my apartment on the other side of the city, but sometimes, when she's inspired to go to class the next day, we're forced to sleep at her place because her campus is practically right across the street. When I ask her why she lives the way she does, she only shrugs her shoulders. It is like asking a bird why it migrates. She is migratory. She will detect a subtle something in the air, a shift in the quality of light that tells her it is time for a change; in the meantime, she does what she feels.

Her bedroom has one small window that looks out over an alley. On summer nights we listen to the hissing gush of vagrants pissing below. The sound of smashing glass is also a common occurrence. I ask her to please not walk through the alley alone. I say: you're the toughest chick I know. It's really the bums I'm trying to protect—trying to protect from your fierceness. And then I squeeze her tiny bicep muscle. I know she does it anyway, though— walk down the alley alone. She's willful like that.

Her nightstand is a stack of books beside the bed, weird books too; weird in the way that if you were trying to guess the kinds of books she reads just by looking at her, you'd probably be way off. Her reading lamp is a single filament light bulb attached to an orange extension cord that runs the entirety of the apartment, down three flights of stairs, and into the back room of a convenience store next door. I ask how long she's been "borrowing" electricity like this and she says: for a while now. This means, as long as she's lived here, or over a year. Single filament bulbs cast perfect shadows. At night we lie in her tiny bed and make shadow creatures on the warped, plaster walls.

When I kiss her, her mouth tastes like cloves. It's got something to do with her chemical composition. I've never experienced anything quite like it. When I kiss her, her mouth is spicy and warm and fully animated. When I kiss her, her fingers go all fidgety. When I kiss her she stands on her toe-tips, and I dip down a little, and our belt buckles click. When I kiss her the awful apartment fades away. I try to kiss her as often as possible.

One morning we awoke to the hum of a cicada-killer hornet trundling sleepily across her dusty hardwood floor. I reached for a sneaker, preparing to attack, and she woke up just enough to say: That's my grandma. Please don't kill her.

How could I have dreamt of killing the hornet grandma she was dreaming of?

I felt something like guilt, something turning toward rottenness deep down inside of me. I wanted to ask for forgiveness, but I didn't know how to, or for what. The whole thing made me feel quiet all day.

You can fuck someone you love, but you don't always love someone you fuck. I love to love to fuck her. I fucking love to love her. When we make love she sometimes puts her hands behind her, on the wall behind her head, and her upside down hands meet at the thumb and forefinger and make the shape of a heart. I love that. She makes the noises her body means for her to make, nothing contrived, nothing theatrical, but nothing repressed either.

It's weird making love to her with her roommates milling about all the time. Sometimes, afterwards, we'll both be in the mood for horchata, and when we leave her room her roommates will look at us like: we know what you were just doing in there. And we'll look back at them

like: that's your problem, pervos. I love feeling like we're in on the same joke.

Probably the only reason to like her apartment is that in the summer it's always colder inside of it than it is outside. It makes her want to snuggle. We've come back from the beach, and on more than one occasion she's replaced her bikini with thick socks and this blue v-neck sweater that used to belong to her grandpa, or someone's grandpa, I don't know. It might be my favorite outfit of hers, the blue sweater with the socks and nothing else. And I do mean: nothing.

I dream secret dreams about her. Secret in the sense that, if I told her about them, she would suspect me of being someone other than the man I've told her I am. I dream of buying her a big house with motion-sensing lights in the yard, and awnings, and porticos, and cedar-lined closets. I dream of filling the hollow, concave space between her hip bones with big, fat babies. Babies everywhere. I dream of life insurance; life insurance paperwork with her name penned on the line for Sole Beneficiary. I dream of her full name remade by my last name.

The erotic dreams, though, I always tell her about. Sometimes I even embellish them. It makes her eyes go goo-goo. If I dreamt we were standing naked in the shower together, I might instead tell her that we were standing naked together in the shower, and that all of a sudden her butchy track coach from high school was there, watching us salaciously through the clear plastic curtain. If I dreamt we were making love in my bed, our bodies dappled by the streetlight coming through my window, I might tell her instead that we were in a nightclub, in the coat check, about to be caught any second. Makes me seems more scandalous than I am. Puts her in the mood, or something.

I tell her little lies that don't do any harm, but there are a few truths I'm keeping tucked away for the time being. I haven't told her I that love her, when I've loved her all along. For now I'm keeping it cupped and covered, like holding a little bird. She is my willowy, wispy girl. I get afraid that the force of my love might blow her away.

THINGS I FIND TO BE CUTE OR HIGHLY ANNOYING

MICHAEL KOH

Annie twitching while sleeping

Annie drooling while sleeping

Annie making strange noises while sleeping

Annie slapping me while sleeping
Annie wrapping her arms around me while sleeping
Annie mumbling while sleeping
Annie kicking me while sleeping
Annie hogging the covers while sleeping
Annie falling off the bed while sleeping
Annie moving close to my body while sleeping

Waking up next to Annie to find out that she is still sleeping

DERRICK MICKELSON'S CUDDLE BED FOR WAYWARD BOYS

TIM JONES-YELVINGTON

Derrick tells me it's wrong to live for him, that I shouldn't live for another person. "What else should we live for," I ask, "if not other people?"

"Live for yourself," he says. "For the things you love to do."

The things I love to do? Biking, blogging, television, jacking off. Great, I think. I'll live for hobbies.

Picture us on opposite sides of the bed, turned toward either wall. The space between us is gravity in reverse. I used to think Derrick's was the coziest bed in the world, but that was before I slept in it every night for two and a half years and it became just my bed.

I told Derrick that I don't need to drink, that I'd be happy giving it up for him, that he's well worth the sacrifice, but he said he shouldn't be the reason I stop.

When Derrick was 14 years old, he raided his parents' liquor cabinet and mixed gin and tonics. One night, after several weeks of this, he stood in his living room and watched his father, a heavy drinker, asleep on the sofa, his arms and legs splayed, his chest rising irregularly, his sleep disturbed. Derrick thought about his childhood, how his father was sometimes himself and sometimes not, and how you never knew which you were going to get. He circled his straw through his drink, displaced ice cubes. He sipped. He said to himself, I could get used to this. Then he emptied his glass into

the bathroom sink. This was 26 years ago, and Derrick hasn't touched alcohol since.

Yesterday, I biked home blackout drunk. I walked in the door just after 6 AM with a bloody lip and ripped, muddy jeans, my bike seat stuck at a 90-degree angle and the shift cord severed. Now Derrick and I are having a "very serious conversation." We're one of those couples that values communication. Generally, "don't go to bed angry" is a good rule to follow. At other times, all I want to do is disappear into the bathroom, lock the door, run a bath, pour essential oils into the water, and play calming music, the kind I would never admit to owning, something categorized by retailers as "adult contemporary," and at these times I wish we were a more normal couple, the kind who might scream and stomp and throw and break things, begin to ignore one another, pass nights with one partner sleeping on the couch.

"I need you to tell me what you're going to do," Derrick says. "To ensure this doesn't happen again."

It's a trick question. If I say I'll never drink again, Derrick won't believe me. If I say I'll moderate my intake, he'll say, "That's what you said last time. You don't know how."

★ ★ ★

Last night I worked a closing shift. I'm employed part-time by Crate and Barrel, selling mass-manufactured housewares. When I visit friends, I recognize their vases, dinnerware, couches. I call them by their names: Good to see you, Birgitta Goblet.

Yesterday I shared a counter with Donna, a woman who tells me stories about douches in the 70s and cocaine in the 80s. I've always taken her lined skin and bleached split ends as signs she's truly lived, and her raspy voice and rattling cough seem to authenticate her experience.

"You wanna know what women want, Benny?" she said.

I expected her to say something expected, something sitcomesque, like multiple orgasms, a deep tissue massage, a man who does as he's told.

Instead, she said, "We wanna get drunk. You coming across the street with us after work?"

As with most of my co-workers, Donna and I have little in common save booze. Across the street from our store is a Mexican restaurant called "Hacienda," but nobody calls it that. We only ever call it "across the street." It's not a real Mexican restaurant, but rather a middle-brow, Tex-Mex chain restaurant-type Mexican restaurant, with papier mache toucans and women in starched, dry-cleaned peasant blouses. I've never tasted their food, only their drinks. They painted a sign on the side of their building—"Es Tiempo por un Swirl!" A Swirl consists of frozen margarita swirled with frozen sangria. They look girly and innocuous, but three of those things will put you under the table.

Last night, I was on my fourth Swirl when I looked at my watch and realized it was already eleven o'clock, the time I'd told Derrick I'd come home when earlier I'd phoned him after closing.

"Time for me to go," I said, sliding off my stool.

"No!" Donna said, then thwumped my back. "Stay with us, Benny. What 23 year old calls it a night at eleven?"

"Ben's married," said Melinda, a fellow sales associate. "His man's got him whipped."

"What?" I said. "That's bullshit."

I called Derrick.

"I'm going to stay out a little longer," I said.

"Okay," he said. "How long?"

"Only an hour or two," I said. "I don't want to get home any later than one."

"I'm going to bed in the next hour. I had a long day."

I tried to read his voice. He sounded okay, like maybe before I called, he'd already resigned himself to an evening alone. I told myself not to worry.

"I'll call you when I'm on my way home."

"How many drinks are you going to have?"

I eyed my fourth Swirl, two thirds of which I'd already downed. "No more than three," I said.

"How many have you had so far?"

"I'm on my second."

"So how many more?" he said.

"One," I said. "Only one."

"How many total?"

"Three," I said. "Only three."

"You promise?"

"I promise."

"Call my cell phone when you're coming home. I'll turn it off when I go to bed so you won't wake me."

★ ★ ★

Before I go any further, I should back up, I should say more about Derrick. So far, you might be inclined to think of Derrick only as uptight, a killjoy. You'll be unlikely to sympathize with Derrick, unless you happen to be Derrick himself, in which case you will say, "I identified with Derrick, and I didn't appreciate how the narrator dismissed Derrick's perspective. The narrator's drinking alienates me like it alienates Derrick. Imagine sitting at home, waiting for the narrator, worrying about his safety. Imagine too doubting the future of your relationship, of your own happiness. Imagine being Derrick's age and still having to cope with such uncertainty."

I met Derrick the same week my mother kicked me out of the house. I met Derrick at church. I didn't attend this church for very long, and neither did Derrick. This church was comprised primarily of homosexuals, their friends and family. The greater denomination of which this church was a member did not approve of homosexuals, and so the church understood theirs as an activist stance.

"I feel too comfortable here," Derrick said after a time. "I feel like we are complacent."

The church held a worship service where the pastor struck a ceramic chalice against the altar and split it in half. The pastor held up the two fragments and said, "These fragments represent our denomination's broken promise. Our denomination has broken Christ's covenant with us through its exclusionary policies. We will not reunite these fragments until these policies have changed."

Then we prayed.

Derrick said, "They are worshipping their own oppression."

Thereafter, Derrick and I spent our Sunday mornings in bed playing pornographic hangman.

"E!" Derrick once guessed. "L! ... T! ... Fellatio!"

When Derrick ran out of guesses, I drew a hanging man with dangling testicles and penis, an X for one eye and a dash for the other.

"His name is Chad," I said.

"Poor Chad," I said. I caressed the paper with my palm. "Sweet hanging Chad."

We nicknamed our bed "Derrick Mickelson's Cuddle Bed for Wayward Boys," a playful reference to Derrick's predilection for caretaking.

Even though we've shared the bed for almost three years, Derrick still likes to place his body in its center, stretch his arms and legs to each side and say, "My bed. Mine."

"Not your bed," I say. "Our bed."

"I bought this bed long before I met you," Derrick says. "This bed has been good to me."

Then he pulls the sheets and blankets up around his face and says, "Swaddle me," and I dive beside him and cuddle him close, thrilled by the reversal of roles.

Derrick taught me things, functional things, like how to balance a checkbook, correctly position a collared shirt on an ironing board, or enhance the flavor of hamburger patties using barbeque sauce and French onion soup mix. I am not the first younger man he's fallen for, and this is something else he taught me, how sometimes it's the younger one who holds the power, on account of we don't necessarily know who we are or what we want, and so we might leave at any moment. When Derrick told me this, how he'd been left, I made a vow never to leave him, because I hate being predictable, and also because I wanted to give him something nobody else ever could.

★ ★ ★

After I got off the phone with Derrick, I texted my friend Miguel: What R U Up 2?

He texted back: Chillin @ home

I responded: Can I cum over?

Miguel works at the store. When I first met him, he didn't make much of an impression, but then a few weeks later, he got a haircut, and I started noticing him. He stood behind the counter as I walked toward him across the sales

floor, and I smiled, and then he smiled back, and the way he smiled, the smile he smiled, that smile hooked me, and that's when I knew I wanted to have sex with him.

We had our first conversation shortly thereafter, in the break room, over lunch. He told me he was a deejay, that he dropped out of college several years ago but wanted to go back, and this time major in sound production. He said someday, after he met the right man, he wanted to raise a kid, but he'd just gotten out of a long, toxic break-up and it was still difficult to trust people. I have always appreciated people who open up about their toxic breakups first thing after meeting you, and so I liked Miguel immediately.

This is where I should probably explain Derrick knows all about Miguel. We have an open relationship, but only when one of us is out of town. Sex only, nothing like prolonged emotional intimacy, everything shared with one another, and I'll be honest—I resent having to explain this, I resent that I can't just say "open relationship" and leave it at that. But I know that if I do not explain, you might misunderstand the situation, and in this case, to misunderstand is to miss the point entirely. Being open brings Derrick and me closer. We check out men together, call attention to those we know the other will appreciate. Sharing fantasies is a bonding ritual, it energizes our sex life. I've never understood why straight couples manufacture such drama by hiding their attractions to others. To ignore these desires, I believe, allows poison to seep slowly into a relationship.

I waited until Derrick was away on business, and then propositioned Miguel in writing, over Facebook. He wrote back, "I think I'm interested but let's talk about it tomorrow."

I prepared our apartment for his visit. I swept and vacuumed and hid the dirty dishes in the oven. I pictured Miguel on top of me and got hard. I wanted to feel his soul patch graze my lower lip, wanted him to look into my eyes and moan my full name, "Benjamin, Benjamin, Benjamin," or even better, its Spanish pronunciation, which sounds like, "Ben ha mean, Ben ha mean, Ben ha mean."

The next day at work, I watched him. I have always been attracted to boys with ADD. Miguel could only hold a conversation for a minute or two before something—a cute child in a stroller, a puppy in a handbag, a well-built heterosexual man on the arm of his fiancée—distracted him. He ricocheted across the sales floor like veggies in a wok, and I would've liked nothing better than to hold him steady.

That night, after our managers dismissed us and he still hadn't said a word to me, I approached him as he opened his locker and said, "Do you have a minute?"

We stood in the rug aisle for what felt far longer than a minute, occasionally looking at one another, but saying nothing.

I giggled.

"What?" he said.

"What what?"

I thought for sure he wanted it, but was perhaps too shy. Derrick once told me single people have more to risk by hooking up with someone partnered, and so they often need the partnered person to make the first move.

"Do you want to come home with me?" I said.

"Listen," he said. "It's like I know myself, right? Sometimes I have these intuitions, like the timing isn't right, or I can feel something isn't a good idea."

I went home, feeling like one of the large rugs had rolled off the shelf and landed on my chest.

As it turned out, that evening in the rug aisle was only the first of many times I did not have sex with Miguel. Later, there was the time he texted me when he knew Derrick was out of town, and said, "Can I come over?" But I'd already jacked off, so I said, "Maybe another time." Or the time I invited him out with me and a friend of ours, but he cancelled at the last minute and said he was staying in, and asked me did I want to stay in with him, but I couldn't think of a polite way to extricate myself from our friend, and so I said, "I'll call you later."

"I know he wants me," I told our mutual friend Cyndi over beers. "Not knowing isn't what bothers me. It's never hearing him say it. It's longing, like in the old days, like we're star-crossed or something. It's good drama, not bad drama."

"If I tell you something, do you promise to vault it?" Cyndi said.

"Vaulted," I said, and made a motion with my fist like I was spinning the dial on a safe.

"Miguel told me he's afraid to hook up with you because you're the kind of person he can see himself falling for."

After that, I became truly obsessed. I needed to hear him say it, hear him say he was afraid of falling in love with me. Or perhaps even make him fall in love with me. I wanted a brief and passionate affair. I wanted to feel tempestuous and torn. Then, after weeks of pitched emotion, I wanted to say to Miguel, "I'm sorry, it's over, my heart still belongs to another." I wanted to put my hand on his chest, kiss his forehead and say, "We'll always have Crate."

★ ★ ★

I took a cab to Miguel's apartment and left my bike chained outside the store. When I got there, he was waiting on the curb, looking intense and revolutionary in an olive commie worker cap, white wife-beater, and one of those Palestinian liberation scarves-turned hipster fashion must-haves draped around his neck. He was shorter than me but also broader, stockier, darker, hairier. He maintained a permanent scruff because he claimed shaving gave him ingrown hairs. I had no idea whether he'd ever cracked the spine on a book of poetry, yet I imagined him dragging his cheek across my nipple while murmuring Neruda.

"Go on inside," he said. "Door's unlocked. I'm going to go grab some beer."

We popped Coronas and sat in front of his laptop. "Have you seen this yet?" he said, and called up a music video on Youtube, a band of shaggy boys with synthesizers, day-glo warpaint on their cheeks.

"Wait," he said. He paused the video a minute in, opened his iTunes. "Have you heard this one?"

Certainly, you must understand why I found him entirely adorable. He was a total spaz, and all I wanted was for him to spaz me. I needed to spaz out.

"It's hot out," he said. He threw his scarf across the tiny room where it landed draped across his sink. He peeled off his top. He unbuttoned his shorts, shimmied and kicked them aside. He grabbed my belt buckle and pulled. "Take these off," he said.

We stood a foot apart in our underwear, drank multiple beers, bobbed casually to the songs on his computer. Women belted rhythmically about the allure and alienation of nightlife. The ceiling light glared; you could see dust bunnies under Miguel's desk. I sucked in my gut, rolled back my shoulders, crossed my arms. I felt a draft and shivered.

Probably, you are wondering about Derrick, whether I gave him any thought. The more sensitive among you might picture Derrick alone in his cuddle bed, sleeping fitfully, awaking periodically to check for me, to wonder when or whether I'll come home.

He'll understand I needed to see this through, I told myself. He'll understand if I'd called him, it would have interrupted the moment. He'll be proud I overcame my fear of initiating, that I finally put this Miguel situation to bed. Got Miguel to tell me everything. Every fucking thing. And then when I come home, I'll bring a sexy story.

"I used to think about you a lot," I said, raising my voice to be heard over the music. "But lately I haven't. Maybe I'm getting over it...You... It."

Immediately, Miguel kneeled, pulled down my briefs, whipped out my dick and stuck it in his mouth. I was flaccid, could almost feel it shrinking inside him.

I should clarify I like blowjobs, but I hate them when I'm not already hard, when I haven't worked up to them, haven't felt a tongue inside my mouth or breath across my neck. And I hate watching them, I always skip that part of any porn film, hate how robotic they look, no bodies touching, no eye contact, like the men are just tools instead of people, like they could be anybody. I feel demeaned, and then I feel embarrassed, and I wonder what's wrong with me for not wanting to watch this, like maybe I'm more like a chick for wanting a bunch of vanilla touching, and then I grow more self conscious, more uncomfortable in my skin.

After a moment, Miguel took it out of his mouth and said, "I like dick."

"I always thought it would be cool if it was like this," he said. "Like you could come over occasionally, no strings attached, we could just get our rocks off."

I reached for another beer and realized the pack was empty. I shook it.

"You got anything else?"

Miguel emptied his cabinets and found a half-empty bottle of cheap Vodka. I grabbed ice from his freezer and filled my glass more than halfway before topping it off with Coke. I thought, tonight might be my last chance. I remembered how in the past alcohol made me more pliable, more willing. I drank.

Miguel sat back down in front of his computer, and I pulled up a chair beside him. I moved closer, wrapped an arm around him, balanced my chin on his shoulder. I felt somehow we'd lost ground. I didn't understand how we went from sucking back to sitting. What was he thinking? I waited for him to make a move, to grab me, move me, take me, take control, to take over, to do *something*. I drank.

Sometime later, he threw open the door to his back porch. We heard birds and saw a hint of sunlight.

"Fuck," he said. "Do you know how late it is? You should go."

I motioned toward his bedroom. "I can crash here."

"I've got a twin bed," he said. "I can't share that shit."

I stared at the wall while I put my clothes on. Once on the corner, I hailed a cab. Halfway home, I drove my fist into the seat. In the rearview mirror, I saw the driver eye me suspiciously.

"Fuck," I said aloud. "Fuck fuck."

What the fuck, I thought. What the fuck was that?

I dialed Miguel's number and his voicemail answered.

"Fuck you," I shouted. The cab driver pulled over, stalled. "I'm sick of this fucking bullshit. You fucking asshole. Fuck. I'm fucking done. Fuck."

I hung up.

"Out," the driver said.

On the curb, I shivered, had a vague recollection of having just yelled into Miguel's voicemail. I immediately dialed his number.

"I think I just said some bullshit," I said. "I'm sorry. I'm coming back down there."

This ends tonight, I thought. Enough. I will make him tell me everything, whatever it takes, however long I have to stand in his apartment, I will make him tell me exactly how he feels about me. I'll tell him what Cyndi said. I'll tell him what I already know. Then he'll tell me. I'll make him.

I hailed another cab. I gave the driver Miguel's address.

A tall, wrought iron fence flanked Miguel's building. The gate was locked. I wrapped my hands around the bars and shook it. I stretched

my leg to the highest crossbar and hoisted myself up, felt the pointed fence top poke my buttock before I landed in a squat, feet throbbing.

The door to Miguel's apartment was behind another locked door. No buzzer. I phoned him again. No answer. I went to the side of the building, pulled up a trashcan, looked in his window. The lights were off, but the glare of his laptop escaped through his open bedroom door into the outer room. Maybe he was awake, watching a movie. I rattled the screen. I banged on the window, lightly, then loudly. I shouted his name.

I heard the front door open behind me. I heard a dog barking somewhere, behind another closed door.

"What are you doing here?" Miguel said.

"I don't... I left..." I couldn't remember.

"You need to go home," he said. "God, are you okay?"

He grabbed my arm, pulled me back through the front gate to the sidewalk. "We need to call you another cab."

"Let go," I said. I pulled my arm free.

I ran. Somewhere, I stopped running, and remembered my bike. Even though the sun was up, I thought, if I leave the bike out all night, it will get stolen.

I do not remember going back to the store, retrieving my bike. I remember riding, how I tore around a corner, through an alley, decided to ride on the sidewalk, caught my wheel on the curb, fell.

I remember later, I looked up, read a street sign, recognized the names, miles north and west of home, I'd taken the wrong street, a diagonal street, and overshot.

I remember I turned, lost my balance, fell. I got up, lost my balance, fell again. I saw my front light bust off the handlebars, heard it scatter across the pavement. I rode. My gears wouldn't shift. My seat was all wrong.

I rode and rode, only sporadically remembering. I remember I saw a familiar train station, realized how much further I still had to go, and I remember I shouted, "I just want to go fucking home, fuck, I just want to go home," and drivers in their cars turned to look at me.

When I opened the door, Derrick was already awake, getting ready for work.

"I'm fine," I said.

"You're bleeding."

"I'm fine."

Derrick held me. He wiped the blood from my lip and fixed me toast with raspberry jam.

★ ★ ★

Now we're lying feet apart at either edge of Derrick Mickelson's Cuddle Bud for Wayward Boys.

Derrick asked me what I was going to do to "ensure this won't happen again," and I told him the accident was a wakeup call, that it traumatized me as much as him. I told him this to keep him from ending us, but also because it might be true.

Then Derrick said maybe we should separate, and I said aren't there other options, and he said, what other options, and that was several minutes ago, and we've been quiet ever since.

The bulb in the fixture above our bed flickers.

"We should buy light bulbs," I say.

"Maybe Lisa has extra," I say, when Derrick doesn't respond. Lisa is our landlord.

"Lisa thinks we should have a ceremony," I say. "She wants to plan our reception."

"I don't need other people to validate my relationships," Derrick says.

"Yeah," I say. I stare at the flickering bulb. "Plus straight people's marriages all end in divorce anyway, right?"

Derrick is quiet again, so I keep right on talking.

"And the ones that don't end in divorce end in death. You either break up or you die. There aren't a lot of options."

The bulb flickers to black. Then it flickers back on, fainter than before. I think about what I want to tell Derrick but can't. How earlier, when he held me, when he pressed the warm washcloth against my cut lip, I could feel what he felt, his terror and relief, and for a moment, I felt happy. I felt happier than I'd felt in ages.

WHAT HE KNOWS ABOUT HER

NATALIE EDWARDS

The woman told him, "I can't be nice tonight."

He said that was fine, and then walked her to his apartment.

In the morning, after she left, he used a lint roller to remove both his hair and hers from the newly washed sheets. His were plenty, dark and curly from all over his body. They seemed woven into the fabric of the bedding. She left fine blond strands. He imagined that only the thinnest, clearest of her hairs would remain— wisps from where her hairline met her temples, feathery arm hair, remnants of the clear trickle under her belly button.

He remembered telling her, "This isn't a thing," and she told him to lie down. He remembered leaning in for the first kiss, and how it wasn't clumsy, but soft. The kiss was like others with women he had waited to kiss so that he might get it right. He tried to recall what she wore, but could only remember her bra, which clasped in the front. It was black and sturdy. He remembered and was embarrassed by the moment when he put his penis close to her face and she didn't take it.

He wondered what color her eyes were. He thought about whether she came and whether or not she put her number in his phone. He recalled her laughing while they were in bed, not a giggle and not a laugh that made him self-conscious.

Based on what he could remember, the woman, from what he could tell, wasn't not nice.

WE CANNOT BE MORE THAN WE ARE

ROXANE GAY

When he comes over, sometimes, he goes directly to the bedroom, kicking his shoes off, emptying his pockets. He carries all manner of things in his pockets—phone, car keys, wrinkled business cards, a lighter because he smokes. There's a familiarity that is irritating.

He throws himself onto my bed on my side and the bed groans because it is eighteen years old. He finds the remote control in the nightstand and starts watching programs I hate. Hockey is stupid. I have to be in love to tolerate a man who watches sports and especially hockey, which is ice soccer, and there is enough ice outside because this is the winter when the world has been shrouded in a thick layer of ice. I don't want to see ice while I am inside. I also don't like Fox News. He would know these things about me if I bothered to tell him. He tucks his hand beneath the elastic band of his boxers and then touches my remote control. When my mother goes to a hotel room, she immediately takes an antiseptic wipe from her purse and begins wiping down everything but especially the telephone receiver and remote control. "You have no idea who has touched these things," she says. I understand, now, what she means.

I go into the living room or my office so I don't say something petty. I don't like to be unkind. I listen to him laughing when he changes the channel to Comedy Central. He always seems to laugh at the wrong parts. Sometimes, we drink wine I consider cheap and he considers fancy. We sit on my couch and watch movies and he says what he thinks I expect him to say about

what he thinks of me—I'm funny, smart, pretty. I have never asked what he thinks of me. I expect nothing from him. He finds it hard to believe I don't need from him what the other women he has known need from him. He thinks I'm laying an elaborate trap where someday, I will change the rules, have expectations. I suppose I should say he hopes. When he tries to say something nice or something implying a future, I tell him to stop talking. I say it politely. I am not rude, but I don't want him to be nice to me. I don't have him over to be nice. Often it is easier to distract him in other ways. He is rather fond of my mouth.

He takes his shoes off and puts his feet on my coffee table. I eat meals on my coffee table and when I eat, I now imagine his feet on my coffee table. It is upsetting. He sits on my couch in his boxers. His legs are pale and hairy, thin. I like being able to hold the remote control, but when he comes over, he assumes the remote control is his purview. That is an annoying masculine trait. He often manages to change the channel at the exact moment when I am starting to enjoy whatever we're watching. There's a show called Snapped on one of those women's cable channels. I get it that there's a moment, often innocuous, when the bough breaks.

Sometimes, he asks, "What are you doing?" I say, "Working." Working is a term that encompasses all manner of computer-related activities rarely related to actual work. I'm writing a paper for an upcoming conference and when he asks about it, tries to show some interest, I offer to let him read it because I know it is boring. He stares at the screen for a few minutes, all those multisyllabic words I am parroting, and says, "Oh," and I take my laptop back. I do not share my real writing with him. He knows I write, but I am vague, I make him think it's a girlish hobby. He found the bookshelves where I keep the books and magazines where I've been published under names that are not my own. He started reading a story I wrote in a book with a racy cover on it. He blushed as he read, deep red streaks shooting from his ears through his neck. He said, "This is great stuff," and I said, "I have no idea where I got those," not because I'm ashamed, but to know my writing is to know me.

I go for days at a time without speaking to him. I tell myself, "I will never see him again." The nights, though, are cold and lonely. He'll send me a text and I'll wait and he'll send another text and another with inappropriate messages of an adult nature, and I'll text back and seven minutes later, there's a knock at the door. When I answer the door, I press my face to the glass and stare at him. He is very good looking. I hate how that makes me feel, how it makes me feel triumphant. I ask him for the password and he says something filthy. My neighbors are likely scandalized or they would be, but many of them are old and hard of hearing.

He likes to keep my wine glass full as if he believes if I drink enough, I'll become different,

warmer, softer, that I'll be open to changing our circumstances. There's not enough wine in the world. I do not require the pretense of conversation or comfortable silence, but he does. He has, in his head, an idea of who a good man is. He wants to be a good man, a good man who treats women respectfully, who wants more than just what "men want." I tell him I don't need him to be a good man, but he cannot hear that. I encourage him to date and even wrote his profile for an online dating site. He showed the profile to me in a previous incarnation and I said, "Unacceptable." It made me sad. There were misspelled words and a terrible picture. I told him to leave me alone for a few minutes. I needed to concentrate. I changed each data field to reflect a better version of him, one that doesn't really exist, but that's what everyone does on the Internet. Everyone deserves happiness.

He goes on dates with local girls, takes them to restaurants and eats loaded potato skins or fried fish or double cheeseburgers. Sometimes there's drinking, beer from the tap, or a movie or, if it's a real special date, a drive out to the closest real town, fifty miles up the road. After these dates, he texts me and comes over and tells me about the dates, the girls, where they ate, what she looked like, what they talked about. He tells me if they made out. He tells me he won't cross the line, and that he knows there's a line even though there isn't. He shows me pictures because my habit of photographing everything is contagious. He tries to make me jealous which

makes me sad, a little, because it doesn't. I tell him, "You're not the only one in my life," and he says, "I have home court advantage," which, I suppose, is true. Anyone I love lives far beyond my reach.

Sometimes I get a phone call and I go on my balcony to talk or into my office. I close the door. When I return, he is stiff, closer to unkind. He answers questions with sharp, one-word answers. He says, "I'm going to go," and I say, "Okay," and he sulks, sinks lower into the couch, his arms crossed over his chest so I'll tap his shoulder and I'll lean down, and I'll whisper in his ear. I'll tell him about all the things I am willing to let him do to me with my hand pressed against his chest, and slowly, he'll relax and I'll feel the slow, steady beat of his heart against my palm and he'll become a bit of a bad man, the kind of man I prefer him to be—a man who is not gentle or patient or kind, who takes what he wants from me how he wants. That's when we get along the best or when I appreciate him the most.

He has used my bath towel, which normally hangs on the end of my bed. He knows where the guest towels are but insists on using my towel. My bed used to be a canopy bed, but I have moved many times and with each move, fewer pieces have made it to the new destination. I suppose the same could be said for myself. When he wants to shower, I offer him the guest bathroom and he says, "Yours is fine." He misses the point completely. There's a familiarity with him that is unearned.

He asks, "Do you want me to stay over?" He keeps waiting for my answer to change. It won't. When he falls asleep, I wonder how long I should wait before waking him up. There are no rules for this sort of thing, but it would be nice if there were. I say, "I have to teach in three hours," and he gets irritated and says, "My leaving won't change that." Sometimes I poke his arm while he sleeps, hoping to rouse him. Sometimes I think he is pretending to sleep but is really awake hoping. He works out, a lot. I am surprised by the thickness of the muscle in his arms and then I'm not because I have seen him apply his strength. He is stronger than I initially realized, a bit of a miscalculation on my part.

When it is getting late, and we're watching television or he is watching television and I am on my laptop *working*, he'll lean back and stretch his arms out like we're in high school. He'll slide closer until our thighs are touching. He'll lean in, and I'll feel his breath on my neck. I will stare harder at whatever is in front of me. He'll put a hand on my thigh or clasp the back of my neck. He might kiss the hollow of my throat or do something less subtle like grab at my breasts or slide his hand between my thighs, pulling them apart. He'll say, "Let's go to bed," as if we're heading in the same direction. I'll know we've pretended to be more than we are for long enough. It is always a relief. I like keeping my bedroom dark, absent of all light. It is an ongoing issue. The temporary blinds I bought fell because the adhesive was weak and

I have yet to find a replacement less tacky than blacking out the windows with garbage bags. In the field outside my bedroom is a tall sign advertising the small community where I live. At night, the light from that sign beams into my bedroom through the curtains. It shines on us, and shows me what we are and what he hopes we will be and everything I don't want from him.

He always lies on my side of the bed and I lie on the wrong side of the bed. It is disconcerting. I feel like I am in a stranger's bed. He likes to kiss. I do too, but not with strangers, so I distract him with things that will make him forget about my lips. He is *very* fond of my mouth. He smiles and touches me gently. He traces my lower lip with his thumb then slides his thumb into my mouth. He likes to talk, to narrate, to remind me of what we're doing. I'm a writer, so he reminds me of what we are doing and I edit, improve his narrative, wish for silence because I am there and I do not require the play by play. I prefer the volume of actions to words. Sometimes, I forget. I forget what we are and are not. I pretend he's someone else, the woman I pretend I'm not in love with because we cannot be different than who we are, the man I'm so in love with and who is so in love with me we cannot let each other go, not really. And yet. We cannot be together, this man and I, because we remind each other of something we've lost, something that mattered more than we understood when we almost had it, her, in our hands. We hurt so much over what we've

lost. We hurt each other. We punish each other. We hold on. When I forget, when the man who is here presses his lips against mine, I don't turn my head away. I open my mouth to his warmth and his tongue and his breath. When we kiss like that, he moans and his voice travels down my throat and I run my fingers through his hair and for small, precious moments, I lose myself or find myself. I cannot be sure. Those moments are terrifying.

When we first met we had a conversation where I was very clear about my interests. I'm older now. The easiest way to get what you want is to ask. He is a small town boy, but he learns fast. I make him blush. I do what I have always done, push push push, see how far I can make a man go. It's a terrible habit, doing that. Someday I'll push too far and I'll only have myself to blame. I've gotten close to too far. I've gotten scared. Sometimes, after, and he hasn't gotten out of my bed yet, hasn't gone home, I close my eyes and I press myself against him and rest my forehead against the back of his neck and I lie very still. If he tries to talk or be sweet, I say, "Please don't. Please don't misunderstand." He always reaches his arm back like he wants to hold my hand. There's that light, you see. I can see his fingers reaching for me, almost trembling. I feel guilty that I allow this thing between us to go on when I know it is going nowhere. I've told him it's going nowhere, but I know he doesn't believe. I lie against him. I reach for him until our fingers are almost touching. I can feel the warmth and imagine how it would be for his fingers to be entwined with mine. I try to wait as long as possible before pushing him away. I love to write stories about girls like me, girls who want everything and will do anything and know nothing.

INTERVIEW: JIMMY PARDO

WHAT HAVE YOU LOST THE MOST SLEEP OVER IN YOUR LIFE?

Jimmy Pardo: Most sleepless nights are spent thinking about four strangers I've had run-ins with and if I ever ran into them again, I would apologize for what I did.

DO YOU HAVE ANY ROUTINES OR REMEDIES FOR WHEN YOU CAN'T SLEEP?

Jimmy Pardo: I spend most of the time doing the pattern in my head of where on the mattress I would end up sleeping if we rotated the mattress at that very moment.

DO YOU HAVE ANY RECURRING DREAMS OR THEMES THAT POP UP REGULARLY?

Jimmy Pardo: Until the day I met the woman who would eventually become my wife, four out of seven dreams would be about running into a girl I hadn't seen since grade school and dating her in present day. The creepy part was that I had no idea what she looked like in the present, so her face would still be the one I knew from back then. As I said, those dreams all ended the day I met my wife.

WHERE'S THE STRANGEST PLACE YOU'VE EVER SLEPT?

Jimmy Pardo: In the record store I managed in the 80s. I went out drinking nearby and was smart enough to sleep with the vinyl rather than drive home

I AM THE SEA CAPTAIN, I AM LANCE ARMSTRONG, I AM TONYA HARDING

ANDREW BALES

Sea Captain

When Ellie finally breaks up with me, I'm still asleep. She doesn't bother to wake me. Instead she has a fully productive day—yoga, brunch, produce shopping, swinging by a FedEx and paying premium for fresh cardboard boxes, returning home to pack her ceramic owl collection—while I'm lost in blank, thoughtless sleep. I wake up to a sharp knocking at the door, and I open it still wearing my boxers. I'm dehydrated and my vision blurs enough that I think maybe it's the mail lady with a package or a broad daylight robbery. I put out my hands as if to say, Take whatever it is you're here for (or) I'll take that package from you.

"Jesus, son, it's three o'clock. Put on some pants," Ellie's father says and lets himself into the living room. Her dad has the wide stance of a foreman and his legs are like untreated lumber forced out of khaki cargo shorts. His polo shirt is tucked in, hugging the beer belly curve, as if he is practicing for yacht club. He flips the shades portion of his glasses up and surveys the living room with his hands on his hips.

"Where are the boxes?" he asks, walking into the bathroom. He leaves the door open, spits in the sink and washes his face. He's using my hand towel to pat himself dry when he pulls back the shower curtains, makes a sour face.

"You've got hard water," he says, returning. "Where are the boxes?"

"Boxes?" I say, and he shakes his head at me.

Ellie's family is new money, still sparkling with novelty. Her parents retired off the settlement they'd made suing a national pet store chain over a rabid bunny. They'd taken Ellie to pick one out for her fifth birthday. She picked a thick white one with bright red eyes, broad saggy ears. She played with it on the floor, named it, imagined her new life with it. She cradled and cuddled and squeezed it until the bunny chomped her cheek, leaving a two-toothed scar down the side. You can't really notice it. Ellie would have to point it out, but she never would. She keeps the groove mortared with makeup, even at home. Learning about the incident was like uncovering a rape. Her recount was a sobbing ordeal with lots of pauses, a mythical tale with phrases like *ferocious fangs*. A story that made you imagine her parents hyping it up in her mind during trial prep.

Ellie's father is staring at our aquarium. He wants to take our fish, he says. He tries to lift it, strains himself until it looks like his back might snap and then he stops. His cheeks turn a little red and his eyes retreat.

"Didn't figure it would be that heavy," he says, as if apologizing. He doesn't ask me to help him lift it, and I'm thankful. "Got Ziplocs?" he asks, staring at the fish with his arms crossed, like they've tricked him somehow. I go to the kitchen and bring back a handful as he begins scooping at them with the little green net.

The fish we had picked out together. In the store—it took weeks for me to convince Ellie to go inside that pet store with me—we walked the perimeter of a dim basement with a few dozen tanks bubbling in a circle around us. I'd picked out a species and then she'd point out the best of the bunch and swipe her credit card at the counter. At home, she loved to methodically feed them. Pinching a few flakes at a time, she'd sprinkle them on the surface and watch from the side with her eyes an inch from the tank, darting back and forth, intently tracking the fish as they swerved and positioned for each morsel.

One by one, Ellie's father captures the fish, plops them into Ziploc bags, and tosses them into a box. Individually packaged in sandwich bags sit our oval rainbow fish, our plump and deformed calico, our transparent glasscat, our heart-shaped discus. One by one, they're stacked until there's nothing left in the tank but plastic shipwrecks on pebbles.

I go to the bedroom to put on pants and I find Ellie's boxes stacked neatly by the chest of drawers. It takes a few rounds of us walking them out to her father's sedan, making only small grunts as we lean in to arrange them in the back seat, before the car's stuffed. I give Ellie's father the flaked food and the aquarium filter. I say maybe I'll give it a few days until I drain the aquarium, give Ellie some time to think it over.

"Don't worry about the tank," he interrupts. "Already got a new one."

Then he shuts the door and is gone.

I sit on the couch with my phone propped on my lap. It doesn't ring. I go to the fridge for leftover pasta salad and find it nearly cleared. There's a little baggie of pasta salad and a note that reads *Needed the Tupperware*. I toss the limp baggie of noodles in the trash. I consider calling, but can't quite bring myself to do it knowing her mom and dad will be there listening, their chins resting upon their fists.

It's mid-afternoon and soon enough it is dusk and then night. I'm in our queen size bed that Ellie's parents found on a hunting trip in Colorado and then shipped the ten hours to Kansas as a surprise for Ellie's first apartment. They bought most things here. The bed is plush and clean. The sheets are blue and gray and contemporary. I lie on my side at first, then diagonally, as if keeping Ellie's space occupied would save us. I shift and flop for hours. From above, I am an X, I am a C, I am an S, I am a whole bowl of alphabet soup dying one letter at a time.

The sea, open and blue. Myself, fitted in a royal coattails getup with accenting white ascot. My sailors, planning revolt, their chests bare and sun burnt and their curly black hairs greasy, knives clenched in their teeth like in the movies. They are hungry, tired, full-on pissed. I could swing across the bow and, in a gentle arc above their heads, anoint each and every one of them with the lavender oil I've been saving for such an atmospheric touch, but instead I bring forth a beat up lawn chair from my quarters and squeak its hinges into position. It's the same aluminum foldout my dad always brought to baseball games when I was ten, before I'd been outgrown by the other boys and was still allowed to pitch. I look nothing like my father. He was lean and tan and strong and dependable in spirit, but even in my deepest dreams I'm pudgy and pale. Even as captain on the high seas I am soft-faced and must clench my teeth to force a strong jaw line for my men. I tell them that I've made mistakes, sure. Who among them might raise his hand and testify that he is without mistakes? Show your hands! When they all raise their malnourished arms, like a pack of bony twigs waving in the breeze, I call on a smaller one in the front. Yes, you, I say.

I sit on the metal lawn chair, the green and yellow weaved fibers creaking, threatening to snap. Not a single mistake to apply to your character? I ask. Of course, Captain, the little man starts. Well, you see then? I say, with my elbows splayed, my palms cradling my head as I recline on the deck above them. I hold out my arms to show sincerity. Everyone makes mistakes! I tell them. But not everyone, a voice calls out from the back, cuts loose a fucking mermaid, sir.

Lance Armstrong

I wake up around noon and spend the day dialing and redialing my voicemail. There are no new messages. I listen to the sterile electronic lady giving me date and time information on month old messages from Ellie asking me to pick up olive rolls or goat cheese, to call her right back, or just five minutes of mistaken pocket noise. I listen to the fabric on her jean pockets swish, the open and closing of car doors, the faint echoes of pop radio and the ticking of turn signals, hoping that somewhere hides a moment of insight, clarity.

If Ellie were here we'd be watching full seasons on Netflix, complaining about other people's decisions or status updates. I try to remember Ellie's favorite flower, color, breed of puppy. I've been too preoccupied for such facts before now. The both of us just out of college, we've finally stumbled into the world we'd been hearing so long about, that looming legend of wholeness and inclusion. The summer is hot and the legend hollow, and two nights ago we found ourselves fighting over which of our friends had better netiquette.

I first met Ellie at a party held on an abandoned floor of a ten-story office building downtown. The place must have been a doctor's office, because there were still boxes of swabs and syringes in the cabinets. The conference room had a long wooden table, but no chairs. Ellie wore bright wristbands that, when taken off and relaxed, resembled the shapes of various cute animals. She took off a panda and gave it to me. We leaned against the table shoulder to shoulder like young business professionals flirting in office catalogs and then sat under the table drinking beers. We were drawn together by fear when some guy stumbled out of the backroom laughing hysterically and bleeding, a dozen syringes hanging from his arms like a dartboard. We became kids running away together from a monster. That night, I later learned, Ellie's family had gone to the country club for a dinner, but she'd escaped. Now, Ellie has finally thought better of it and escaped our life and returned to theirs.

There's knocking. Ellie's father is at the door. He wants more boxes. I try not to look

too beat up about it as we get the last of them in the backseat. Inside, we stand awkwardly. He coughs and looks down at the pea green rug under the coffee table. I move the table to the side and he rolls up the rug and droops it over his shoulder.

I tell him I'm sorry, but I need to know, will she come talk to me?

He puts his hand on my shoulder, a tender touch like a pastor at a funeral might deliver.

I spend the night on the porch drinking beer. It is dusk out, and the cicadas remind me of the vacancy with their drone.

Pumping thick thighs, I am Lance Armstrong, mid-race on some mountain climb in France, hyper-aware that the world is watching. At home, millions of delicate hands fondle my wristbands. Yellow. Smart. Active. Alive. I am taking deep breaths and focusing on my position. My arms. My breathing. My front tire going soft. The rider in front of me resigns himself to this bitch of a hill and rides right off its steep face. Who can blame him? Who chose this hill, forty-five degrees plus? Who designs a course destined for failure? The other riders, skeleton figured men with thighs like hams are strewn along the side of the course, polka dotting the landscape with spandex greens and hot pinks, clutching their calves as they cry out for their managers and sponsors. They cast off their helmets and, losing the thick veneer of sportsman ego, hold each other tenderly and begin to weep. But I push on. I am not destined for failure. Did you see those kids in Illinois with the wristbands? Their swooning eyes? Do you understand? Those kids probably don't even know about the one testicle thing. They are pure. Hope. And for their parents, the husband with honest-to-God one nut, or figurative one nut, who clutches at his wife's wily feet as she leaves him for a new life, as she looks down, disgusted at this dramatic display of neediness after countless years of guarded aloofness, breaks free and gently closes the door behind her. This is why Lance Armstrong peddles into coma, lives strong.

Tonya Harding

Knocking. It's two teen boys this time, and they've backed their pickup across the lawn right up to the porch.

"There's nothing left," I say.

"Jim says to get the bed," the taller one says.

This is how I learn Ellie's father's name.

The shorter one with the square head says that if I put up a fight they've been authorized to start some shit. They're still giggling when I'm back inside in the kitchen. They stalk the bed, circle it, poke at it like it might be a trap. Both of them have buzz cuts and arms with muscles defined by abuse, not athletic care. Their smiles are a little crooked, unsettling.

"Nice bed," the taller one says. "What's this, a queen?"

The little guy winks at me. Says, "You called it."

They giggle.

"Just take it," I say. They flip it up on its side and run it into the door and push it onto the porch. They lift it into the back of the pickup and return to do the same number with the box springs. They knock it against the doorframe, scrape the hardwood floor with its plastic edge. I call at them to lift, but it's too late. The screen door slams shut. They don't turn back, just get in the truck and drive across my lawn.

My house is a stripped car. I still have the frame, but the engine is gone. I lie on the floor in the bedroom inside the metal frame where the bed used to rest. There's no churning from the fish tank in the living room, no scattering of light across the ceiling. The house is empty and still. Ellie is gone and not coming back. Down here it is colder, much colder, and I remember as a kid learning how heat rises and gets trapped with you in the top bunk. I remember the climb and the space that was yours alone. I remember the little TV with the power cord that would just barely reach, catching some stray signal by leaning the antenna against the bed frame. Mining the air for a few lost waves.

I can almost still hear my raspy, commanding voice: If you need a hotel, I can book you a hotel. If you need a flight, a flight. If you need reading materials for said flight, that's a personal expense. I'm a professional and I expect you to be one too. I just, well, you don't need my reasons. I just need this. I need this done right. The two men in front of me nod along, vacant eyes in thick skulls. Did I ever tell you, I ask, that I performed the triple axel jump in competition? I'm the second person ever to pull together such a bird of paradise display. No one cares. The two men look at one

another, then back at me, blinking. Okay. Look, I'm not diminishing Nancy. I'm not calling her a robin or some black-capped chickadee. But you two are hunters by trade, so that makes it all the more worth your while. Here's your money. Go. Find her.

I'm in a gas station on the way home, waiting in line to put ten dollars on three. There's something lonely about the reflection of my frizzy haircut off a Zippo lighter display. I'll get gas and go home. I'll eat a bowl of cereal and get ready for work and get Nancy out of my mind. Work is a boxing ring inside a large metal warehouse. I oversee amateur wrestlers with proud, bald heads. Men of caliber. Entertainers. I stand cross-armed ringside and manage them as they pummel the bejesus out of other men. False swings and throws for the most part, but sometimes they really connect. Everyone knows it happens sometimes, and that's why it takes so much courage. Backstage before the fight, hiding their identity with makeup—the electric blues and lightning bolt whites—smothering their faces

in mixed putty colors with my own hands, whispering in their ear before the match as how to break a chair over someone's head with just the right amount of authenticity, these are my moments. We win titles and tie ourselves together on stage with heavy gold belts. I don't need anyone but them. My fighters and belts. I'm next in line when I see out of the corner of my eye, in the casino area that's roped off with a plastic chain, an old woman falling from her perched position on a stool in front of a video poker machine. The clerk looks over, the customers hush, and then everyone's back to browsing candy bars, looking for barcodes on milk jugs. I step out of line, go over to her, stoop down. The old lady's eyes are closed. Her gray hair in perfect puffball form. I check her breathing. Zilch. I think of health class and lifeguard training in high school. Blank. Then I remember something from TV and pump her chest to the rhythm of "Stayin' Alive." I pinch her nose, breathe into her lungs. Her small chest swells up from the pressure, but she's

staying under. How far gone is she? She's maybe four feet under at this point. Probably at the stage where you get to see yourself being worked over but don't feel too disturbed about watching your body bent and broken. Maybe she can see me stopping to yell at her. I'm inches in front of her face screaming, "Giving up? Giving up now?" I pump her chest with clenched fists. I lean over her, pushing every last bit of myself into her mouth, down through her esophagus, into her chest. I'm absorbed by her body and distributed through her veins via red blood cells. I am a life force in equal measure to how much of a parasite I've been with the rest of my time. I feel her chest ballooning with my breath. I feel these millions of bits of myself ushering her back to life. I feel vindicated, saintly, resolved. I feel like a person who has finally done something right until I hear a pop as her chest explodes like a Chinese watermelon, as her flesh flies forth and hangs from my fingers, my nose, the legs and sandals of standers nearby, the young clerk with an open mouth but nothing to say.

[the fourth house]

J.A. TYLER

I built a fourth house underneath a mountain. The mountain was tall but I moved it stone by stone, tree by tree, displaced its bulk until there was a hole I could stand in. I stood in the mountain's lack and built a house there. This fourth house. I went back to my axe, my saw,

planks from trees and the mud for sometimes seams. I built a chimney for the first snow, gutters for the first rain. I built shelves where the jam would go. I built cupboards for my magic tricks, my deck of cards. I built a closet for my violin, the drippings of its music. I built a corner where I could stand. I built a chair where I could sit. I built a bed to cover in a quilt of pine needles and moss. I built my mother to rock me to sleep and my father to cook up our fish in the mornings. I built a picture frame and a picture of my brother inside of it, to keep track of what was missing.

When I was a child and my brother was a child, we were deer and we ran through these woods, our hooves light with wild, our mouths with mountain air. My brother would dip into the river and I would follow. We would wade. My brother would raise his head to a bird going from branches. My brother would eye a squirrel digging in root systems. My brother would hang his antlers on the sky. I would follow, always behind, my deer-brother and this forest.

In these woods, I am only trying to survive.

These woods, the woods I am in now, these are the same woods that my brother and I would run through, tumble in, but without the life that was there, the youth, the living. I appeared here, in these trees, looking upward at clouds. I don't know how it happened. My brother found me in these woods. I awoke and he was above my body, haloed in sun. Half-brother, half-deer. All-deer and no river. All-brother and this message: *You are dying*.

My deer-brother, in his hand was a piece of paper, on the paper a black dot. And inside of the black dot those remembrances of how our antlers hooked, of how we punched each other in our boy-faces, laughing. And inside of those fists were pictures of us as kids. Inside of everything was this forest, the deer-brothers we are, running.

In these woods, escape is not always attached to hooves.

In this fourth house I made a doorway with no door. Instead I restacked what was left of the mountain, tree by tree, stone by stone, leaving open only a space between the mountain's skin and my heart, so that I was living inside of a cabin inside of a cave inside of a mountain inside of the dying that I was going through, that my brother was professing. The layers of that doorway were dark. And only once did a bear come to find me there, no room left for hibernation, my knife at the ready. The red on the walls from this bear was invisible in our darkness. He was not my brother. I have no bear-brothers.

In the darkness I played at pretend. I pretended I was the sky. I floated. I pretended I was a river. I crossed through myself. I pretended that I was a deer, running beside my brother. I pretended I was in a cabin in a cave in a mountain in a lost woods where I was dying. I pretended I was only sleeping. I pretended that what felt like a bed beneath my body was instead a forest floor, soft earth and hope, light as treading hooves.

In these woods, escape is sometimes pretending.

My brother's hand was trembling when he handed me my death, that paper with such blackness in it. I wanted my brother's trembles to have been his fear at losing me in more than a lost woods. Bedside scarring. I wanted the sun to come up with other bears entering this cabin in this cave in this mountain. I wanted to slit them open, to swim in red, to paint myself in anger, to drip with all these notions of brotherhood. I didn't want to sleep as it is, forever.

In these woods my knife grew meaningless.

In this fourth house, after a decade, the dark proved too much. On every wall was a sky, and in all the skies there were no stars. My brother

never re-appeared, no other bears came, and the blood on the walls dried and I could no longer paint words. There was no longer any secrecy to living in a cabin in a cave in a mountain. There was no longer reason to hide, no one was looking.

In this fourth house, the game of pretend had turned into the game of non-existence, so that everything I imagined was all that didn't belong, until everything in the woods didn't belong and I didn't belong and there wasn't anything left to pretend. I had pretended it all, and nothing was left to admire. It was a darkness unlike any darkness.

Deer-brother, please come light this up.

Sleep is not escape.

I burned the fourth house inside of the cave inside of the mountain. There was no other answer. The flames were monotonous and bright. The mountain sighed back down into itself when the structure deflated, one hollowed bear within, and me walking back into these lost woods.

In these woods I want to undo what has been done. In these woods there are an infinite number of houses to build and burn down. In these woods my brother handed me a note, and the note said my death, and I was lost. In these woods, a hundred bears will never equal a deer-brother, spinning hooves through trees, a way of living.

CRAMPS

ETGAR KERET

That night I dreamed that I was a forty-year-old woman and my husband was a retired colonel. He was running a community center in a poor neighborhood, and his social skills were shit. His workers hated him because he kept yelling at them. They complained that

he treated them like they were in basic training. Every morning I'd make him an omelet, and for supper a veal cutlet with mashed potatoes. When he was in a decent mood, he'd say the food tasted good. He never offered to clear the table. Once a month or so, he'd bring home a bouquet of dead flowers that immigrant kids used to sell at the intersection where the lights were really slow.

That night I dreamed that I was a forty-year-old woman and that I was having cramps, and it's nighttime, and suddenly I realize I'm all out of tampons, and I try to wake my husband, who's a retired colonel, and ask him to go to the all-night pharmacy or to drive me there at least, because I don't have a driver's license, and even if I did, he still has an army car I'm not allowed to drive. I tell him it's an emergency, but he won't go, just keeps mumbling in his sleep, saying the meal was lousy, and that if the cooks thought they were getting furlough, they could just forget it, because this was the army and not some fucking summer camp. I stuffed in a folded Kleenex and tried lying on my back without breathing, to keep it from leaking. But my whole body hurt, and the blood was gushing out of me, sounding like a broken sewage pipe. It leaked over my hips, and my legs, and splashed over my stomach. And the tissue turned into a wad that stuck to my hair and my skin.

That night I dreamed that I was a forty-year-old woman and that I was disgusted with myself, with my life. With not having a driver's license, with not knowing English, with never having been abroad. The blood that had dripped all over me was beginning to harden, and it felt like a kind of curse. Like my period would never end.

That night I dreamed that I was a forty-year-old woman and that I fell asleep and dreamed I was a twenty-seven-year-old man who gets his wife pregnant, and then finishes medical school and forces her and the baby to join him when he goes to do his residency abroad. They suffer terribly. They don't know a word of English. They don't have any friends, and it's cold outside, and snowing. And then, one Sunday, I take them on a picnic and spread out the blanket on the lawn, and they put out the food they've brought. And after we finish eating, I take out a hunting rifle and I shoot them like dogs. The policemen come to my house. The finest detectives in the Bloomington police force try to make me confess. They put me in this room, they yell at me, they won't let me smoke, they won't let me go to the bathroom, but I don't crack. And my husband beside me in bed keeps yelling, "I don't give a goddamn how you did it before. Around here I'm the commander now!"

WHERE ONCE WAS A CLEARING, MORE FOREST

SIMON A. SMITH

For Wilson

When Ralph got home from his support group, the house was warm and inviting, but silent. He was surprised and a little dismayed to find that he was home alone. He had made a breakthrough at the meeting, was feeling balanced and grateful for a change, and he had at least wanted someone around to witness his elevated mood. It had been a monumental task raising his spirits to this modest height and now he was worried that, left on his own, he would lose his will. Just as he felt the deflation coming on he heard Mary, pouring water from the kettle in the kitchen. In the empty stillness of the foyer, the light splash of tea filling a mug sounded like a

large blessing and went a long way in loosening his nerves. Ralph hung his coat in the closet. The new hush in the house was toying with his temperament, threatening his disposition. He didn't know what to expect this evening. For several days, weeks almost, there had been very little communication between the two of them, no affection at all, but at least before there had been the noise of the television at night to keep them company.

Ralph smoothed his hand down the closet door as he pushed it shut behind him. He looked at the narrow hallway leading to the bedroom, the bookshelf at the far end that used to hold

their wedding photo. He'd have to pass Mary and the kitchen on his way to the bedroom, break the quiet with his plodding footsteps. He took a deep breath, moved forward.

Because he couldn't help himself, Ralph slowed when he reached the kitchen and peeked through the open doorframe. He saw Mary standing with her back to him, her fluffy blue robe pulled tight around her waist. Her two pale legs, poking out the bottom, were so sleek and white he worried they might melt so close to the stove. Besides the robe, there was the fatigue that hung on her like a separate garment—the saggy pillows of skin beneath her eyes, the droopy shoulders and wobbly knees.

Ralph slipped through the bedroom door and slid onto the bed. Mary's voice called from the kitchen.

"Would you like some tea?" she asked.

"Okay. Yes," Ralph said.

Mary opened the cabinet and Ralph heard her bring down another mug. He situated himself on the edge of the bed and untied his boots. He removed one boot by hand, then stamped on the heel of the other and pried it off with his wet foot.

"Why is the TV off?" Ralph asked. He heard her pour another sizzling portion of water into his mug. He thought about asking for honey, but decided it would be better not to.

"I thought we'd talk," said Mary.

"Oh?" Ralph said. He straightened his boots, tucked the laces inside, and scooted them against the wall. By the time he looked up, Mary was already upon him, swooping around the corner, handing over his tea and sitting next to him on the other side of the bed. Her sudden presence startled him, took his breath away even. To mask the quick burst of anxiety, he lifted the mug, hiding his face in the steam.

Mary was arching forward on the sagging mattress, cradling her mug in both hands. Over the rim of his own mug, Ralph saw that something significant had changed in Mary since he'd left that afternoon. Something frigid had thawed inside of her, and the runoff had settled in the bottoms of her pink, dewy eyelids. There was compassion in those eyes now, a fresh sense of contentment. Her casual posture, tipped toward him with her elbows resting on her thighs, revealed that she had come to terms with something she'd been struggling against. When she smiled at him, the openness, the unfolding that came with it, made his throat constrict. He swallowed.

"How does it feel to be drinking green tea at six o'clock?" Mary said.

"Odd," said Ralph, and he laughed as he added, "like feeding tomato soup to a car engine. Pointless."

Ralph was pleased when Mary returned the laugh. "Not pointless anymore," she said. "It's a good substitute. Good for your digestion. Medicine, if you will."

"I've had enough caffeine in the past couple of days to keep a whole family awake for weeks.

Anyway… a new kind of medicine is a good way to look at it I suppose," Ralph said. He slurped his tea.

Ralph was still getting used to the renewed sense of comfort between them. It had been weeks since they had been flirtatious with one another, weeks where flirtation would have been impossible. He felt a little shy and self-conscious. He drank his tea and stared out the window across from him. It was getting darker earlier. Winter would be there before they knew it. The tree limbs were turning naked and spindly in the grayish light, stiff from the cold. Ralph reached into the breast pocket of his flannel and brought out some matches and a pack of Camels. He shook a cigarette out and pinched it between his lips. He scooped his hand under the bed, dragged out the glass ashtray and set it by his toes. He lit a match.

In the pause, Mary glanced down at the floor. There, weeping on the wooden surface, were small horseshoes of condensation from Ralph's boots, a trail leading through the door and ending at his discarded footwear. They both stared at them for a moment.

"How'd the meeting go?" Mary asked.

"Okay," said Ralph, snapping out of it. "Joe asked if I wanted to go hunting this weekend up in Michigan." It wasn't what he had planned on talking about, but then he hadn't planned on sitting on the bed next to Mary like this, with her bare legs so close and the whistling

hiss of the radiator filling so much muted space between them…

"Really?" she said. "That sounds nice. Hey, I think that's really nice. That can't hurt anything, right?"

She was taking her time, Ralph thought, wading into things, which he could appreciate. But he couldn't help himself. "I haven't been hunting in a week or so," he said. And already he could feel his erratic mood turning against him. There was nothing he could do about it now. Everything had happened so fast.

"It's been longer than that, hasn't it? It's been over a month, right?"

Ralph put his tea on the bed beside him. He wiped his lips with the top of his hand and kept it there, breathing into his knuckles. After a while he flicked his ash into the tray and took another long drag.

"What is it?" Mary said.

Ralph let the smoke come trickling out his mouth and nose. He was still gazing toward the window but it was a meaningless gaze. His eyes weren't seeing or recording anything. He couldn't focus. He wished he could have prepared himself for this. It worried him that he didn't know what he was about to say.

"Remember how much I used to love hunting?" Ralph said.

"You were a hunting fiend," she said.

"I was obsessed," he said.

"You made me nervous," Mary joked. She

started to laugh but stopped when she saw Ralph wasn't smiling.

Ralph licked his lips, raked his teeth across a cracked spot, and bit down. He took another pull from his smoke. "When I was a kid I couldn't stand hunting," he said. "I hated everything about it. I hated guns. They scared the shit out of me. People who held them, aimed them... I didn't like it when my dad left for a whole week, and I never understood what was so great about shooting some defenseless thing, bringing it home for dinner..." He smashed his butt out in the ashtray and right away plucked out the pack and went in for another. "It made my stomach turn to eat that meat, but I guess I ate it anyway. Course, I didn't have a choice... gun still propped against the table like it was." He lit the cigarette and threw away the match.

"Your dad was a difficult man," said Mary.

"That's a nice way to put it," Ralph said.

"Well, it doesn't mean anything," she said. She reached her arm back and planted her hand on the bed for support, letting her shiny hair spill down over her dipped shoulder blade. She sipped her tea.

Where had this breezy attitude come from? Was she tempting him, taunting him? Ralph wanted to know. He took another drag, chased it with some tea. "Keith was the one who got me hooked. Remember Keith?" Ralph asked.

"Oh, you know I do. Of course I do. Whatever happened to Keith? I haven't seen him..."

"I haven't a clue."

"You guys used to be inseparable," Mary said.

"Unstoppable. We were. I don't remember every detail anymore, but I'm sure it was my fault," Ralph said.

"Don't be like that, now. Now's not the time to be talking like that," she said.

"I can be sure it was my fault, because I made sure of it. I shoved him off. I mean, it was by choice... There were no accidents. I didn't want anyone seeing me, but..." Ralph took a quick puff, exhaled. He shook his head. "Ha! I was *hiding out!*" He said it with the force of regret behind it, like he was scolding himself. The mug flopped about on the bed, murky water spraying out and dotting the sheets. Ralph picked it up, took a sip, and set it on the floor.

"They'll all forgive you. They will," Mary said.

"Keith. Keith was a pretty good marksman, but he was a master field dresser," he said.

"Field dresser?"

"A gut head," he said, "a butcher. Keith used to dress the deer right there in the forest. Most people haul the deer back to a shed, like my dad, and they mount the deer somewheres and slice it up, but Keith didn't need to."

"Oh? I see," said Mary. She pushed herself back up straight, took another sip of tea. Something went off inside of her. Ralph could see that some switch had been triggered. All at once she looked alive, like she'd been slapped awake, and he thought she might be getting it.

"When Keith first taught me how to do it, how to knife into the deer and cut it open—I didn't know what to think. It wasn't me, you know? I didn't rip things open like that, for sport or whatever—for fun. But Keith did. Keith'd get so excited and giddy, you know? He'd be kneeling there in the mud with his tongue out, carving away like a kid in art class and he was just goofing off. It was no big deal. And he made it look fun. He did. A big old smile on his face... It took the edge off... the fear, that hesitancy, you know? It was like he was doing it to music, and he was like, glowing," Ralph said. He chuckled a little, remembering it. He knocked the ash off his smoke and took a heavy pull.

"You guys always seemed so happy when you came back. You brought home a lot of good meat," Mary said. There was a hesitancy in her voice now, a hitch. She was measuring her words, testing them out.

"More than you know," Ralph said. He started to talk again but stopped. He took a deep breath. His words came slow and serious. "Once Keith showed me a bunch of times how to do it, I got really good. I think I might have even been better than him. I was more into it. It was strange. He seemed to take less pleasure in it the more I did. I like, turned into him, and then he turned into me, and I just kept going. I became someone else or something else. I *needed* it more than he did. I couldn't get enough," he said. He took one last puff of his cigarette and stabbed it out.

"The hunting or the dressing?" Mary asked.

"I rented a freezer at one of the campgrounds up there in Pike County. Couple of weeks ago. I had so much meat stacked in there nobody would ever be able to eat it!" He was speeding up, words piling and overlapping one another.

"I didn't know about that," Mary said. She gripped her mug tighter. The color drained from her face.

Ralph looked at her with a crooked grin. "Not later on, you didn't. You didn't know about last month, but in the beginning you knew. Before my Dad died."

And then, in a sudden surge of panic, Ralph saw that Mary knew what they were talking about. He saw the look of shock on her face, could almost see her heart beating faster through the robe. She couldn't get enough tea. She kept nipping at it, pecking at the water the way a bird goes after food. "I went hunting, too, for a while. Is that what you mean?"

"Yes. Yes, you did," Ralph said. "You had your own sort of hunting for a while there. We used to go out together. You were hitting it pretty hard, keeping up. It was pretty fun at first."

"You're talking about years ago, Ralph, before we got married. We were only twenty-two, twenty-three. We were kids. It's fun being wild when you're twenty-three. I'd absolutely insist on it, but..."

"Yes, but you had your reasons even back then," Ralph said. "I could see it. You weren't

just hunting for fun's sake, were you? You weren't eating everything you killed. Ha ha!" Ralph laughed. "That's a good one. You were staying out later than everyone else, me and you... getting back after the sun came up, staying in bed the whole next day with the blinds drawn shut."

"I guess I had my own... reasons, I guess..."

"You had your own kind... your own sort of Dad stuff... You must have..." He stopped, cleared his throat. He softened his voice, talked at the floor. "Not exactly... Whatever your own situations were, only you know... or something," he said. "I should have asked, but we were both in no place for reflection."

"But I didn't know you were doing it like that... the last few weeks, not in that way, not in that kind of state, I didn't know. I thought we gave up that business a long time ago. We talked about it, remember? That's not fair."

"I know," Ralph said. His volume rose. He reached up and yanked down on the side of his head, cracked his neck, twisted his torso. "I guess I never stopped all the way, not like you did. Then, after Dad, the last few weeks, I went nuts. I drove all the way up to Pike County on my own. Keith thought I was crazy. I thought I was crazy too, but then I didn't care anymore. I was lonely at first, but then I got over it. I felt like shit and that just made me want to do it more. My mind was zooming ninety miles an hour. Non-stop!" he said, clapping his hands together, sending each hand bouncing in opposite directions. "You had more control, Mary. You always did. Maybe it was in my genes or something, I don't know. It got to the point where I lost all sense of law and decency. I'd have shot a duck on the first day of summer," he said. "Could have been the day of a birth, probably. A wedding I'm sure wouldn't have stopped me. A funeral..." He slumped forward, rocked back and forth.

"Ralph?" Mary said. She turned to face Ralph, pointed her knees at him. "It's been almost a month since your Dad passed away. Those last few weeks leading up to the driveway incident last Tuesday... the hospital... I must have been the biggest idiot. You must have taken me for a dumb, dumb bitch."

"No. No, Mary. I didn't take anybody for nothing. I had no control over it."

"Why did you do that to me?" Mary said.

"I didn't tell anyone. I was ashamed. My dad would have killed me," Ralph said. His tone changed, downshifted. Some new, somber emotion came flooding in. "Keith didn't understand either. I really wanted him to in the beginning, desperately, but then at the end I was glad he wasn't around to see me."

"I thought you were distraught over your dad. Every time you grabbed another drink from the fridge after work I blamed it on your dad."

"I'm a fuck up," Ralph said. "My dad would have killed me."

"When you stayed up until five in the morning, I blamed it on your dad. I thought

you were grieving. You said you were grieving. You lied to me. When you went into the spare bedroom with your headphones on and you turned the lights off and didn't come out for hours…" There were tears forming in her eyes and she angrily swabbed them away with her finger. "You treated me like I was stupid garbage. You made me feel helpless."

"I was protecting myself. Grieving can look like that. It can look any which way. I've already discussed this once tonight!" Ralph said. "It's a selfish thing, I know that." He couldn't look at Mary. His eyes were still trained on the floor.

"When you got home an hour late from work I blamed it on the fact that you couldn't get up in the morning, because you didn't go to sleep the night before. It was endless, my stupidity." Mary stood up from the bed, leaned in over him the way a mother does to a son. "Do you know how it makes me feel that you couldn't trust me with this? I'm your wife!" she shouted.

"I felt like I was protecting you. That's the space I was in, believe it or not. I didn't tell Keith or you… I'd have only scared you and him and anyone else… I was scared to death of myself!" he said.

Mary straightened up. She sighed, grabbed her hair, mashed it between her fingers. "Ralph. Ralph, you're not a frightening person. You're not like other… hunters… other gunmen you've known." Mary stopped. In the silence, Ralph looked up and followed Mary's eyes with his own. They landed on a photograph resting on

their nightstand. By the alarm clock sat a picture of Ralph's dad in his hunting getup, his bright orange hat, his camouflage vest and his extra long beard. He was kneeling there in the middle of the woods and, stretched across his knee, dangling there, was the still warm carcass of a white-tailed deer with a nine-point rack. It was one of the only photos Ralph ever saw where his dad was smiling. "You've never been like that," Mary said. "You were always the hunted." She turned toward him again, and Ralph could feel her trying to draw his attention, but he couldn't take his eyes off the photo.

"I used to be driving home from work and I'd be talking to myself. 'You're not going to Pike today, are ya? Are ya, Ralph?' I'd be asking myself. 'You just went up there yesterday. You don't need that. Relax. Come on.' And I'd convince myself that I was stable, but then the dialogue would keep going. 'Ah, what's the big deal? Go on up. Go ahead, ya sissy. What's the big deal? Just for a little bit. You'll be fine. So, you need a little break. So what. It's fine. You know you want it. Don't torture yourself like this, for God's sake.' And I'd be gone. I'd get to exit fifteen and I'd still be arguing with myself. Sometimes I'd nearly crash into the guardrail, spinning the steering wheel at the last second, screeching the tires, hitting the exit ramp way too fast, heading north. Every time…"

"You should give Keith a call," Mary said. "Keith loves you. I bet he'd go with you to your meetings. He'd support you."

"After the funeral, I went wild," Ralph said with a disgusted laugh. "Woo-hoo! Keith and I, we used to go for a weekend, and I would look forward to doing it again in a few weeks. I was anxious, but I could wait. Then I couldn't live without doing it every few days, then every day, then three times a day. I couldn't even remember what it was like to not be in the middle of all those trees." Ralph closed his eyes. He clenched his fists and pressed them against his legs. "You keep looking for that light at the end of the darkness, because you know it used to be there. There was that place, you know? Where you used to sit a bit, unwind, catch your breath, take a little rest. But shit, you haven't seen it in… in ages."

"I know," Mary said, and she was crying. Ralph could hear her sniffling. "I know, baby." She reached out to him, and even the action of the reach, the motion, seemed loud, like it made noise, and Ralph flinched when she put her hand on his knee. He kept his eyes closed.

"I can still see those carcasses splayed out on the brush. Those little kidneys. Those lungs. That itty-bitty heart. Part of me hated seeing that heart exposed. I hated that I'd been the one to stop that heart. And my heart was still beating. I could feel my own God damned heart thumping. It'd be thumping so hard. I'd get so angry at myself, sometimes I'd almost forget whose organs I was looking at. I had a sharp knife, boy…"

"Ralph, please," Mary pleaded. Her voice was changing over from sadness to anger. Ralph knew this mode, knew how her temperature could rise in a hurry. Her shoulders would be twitching, her eyes blinking. She snorted.

"I'm sorry, Mary," Ralph said. He opened his eyes and his words started racing again. "Hiding it was the worst part. You didn't know. I used to lay right here in this bed, hating myself." He turned around and ran his palm over the comforter. "I couldn't live with myself. If you hadn't found me out in the driveway, in the truck…"

"I was so angry at you," Mary said, and Ralph could tell that she was mad at those awful tears for still coming. She leaned over and grabbed a tissue from the nightstand.

"I don't even remember waking up…"

"That's because you wouldn't," Mary interrupted, rubbing her nose clean, wiping her eyes with the bathrobe sleeve. "Draped there in the seat, blacked out, pale as a ghost, drooling, bottles everywhere. I thought you were dead!" she yelled. Now her whole body was trembling and she covered her eyes with her hand, clawing at them like she meant to rip them out.

"Medicine bottles," Ralph whispered. "I don't even know how I made it home," he said.

"God only knows," said Mary, shaking her head, trying to reel herself back in.

"The truck knew the way."

"Don't you ever do that again," Mary said. She uncovered her eyes, breathed into her cupped hand.

"I won't," Ralph said. "I won't I won't I won't," he whispered. "No more hiding."

He put his head back and stared at the ceiling. He sensed his eyes growing large, dilating. He bent back, took a huge gulping breath, ran his hands over his eyes and dug his fingers into his cheeks. He jerked straight up, kicking the tea on the floor. It felt as if he'd had a nightmare and been jostled awake. He watched Mary pinch her collar shut. She lowered her head, turned away, clamped her chin against her armpit and wiped her nose there. Ralph hated that she was embarrassed, as if she was the one who needed to shrink from these confessions.

"I'm sorry," Ralph said. "I shouldn't have done that. It's just that we haven't talked for so long and…"

"No," said Mary, sniffling, "you needed to get it out. I must have been begging for it. God, I get so confused about what I'm doing and why…"

A long pause followed. Ralph knew that he should tell her that he wasn't going hunting with Joe, that even though it wasn't the main problem, and he had been working hard on the real, underlying issues, it wasn't time. He wanted to put his arm around her, maybe massage her back. How could he do that now? How could he ever approach her or touch her again? He didn't deserve to. She didn't even trust him enough to let their feet brush together while they were falling asleep anymore. Any second she could

stand up and tell him she was leaving, and he knew he wasn't ready for that kind of letdown yet. Jesus, how did anyone ever know how to react to something like this? Things were never supposed to turn out this way. They'd have to start all over again.

When the phone rang both of them whipped their heads toward where it rested on the desk. The rush of sound, tumbling out of the silence, had given them a jolt. Mary gasped. She was only a few feet away.

"Answer it," Ralph said.

"I don't think I can," Mary said.

"Please," said Ralph.

"I'm not in the right frame of mind."

"Please," said Ralph again, more insistent this time. "Please answer it. This is important."

"Okay," said Mary. She cleared her throat, snorted again. Her eyes were red and swollen. She moaned as she shuffled toward the desk.

Just as she was about to push the button Ralph said, "Whoever it is, tell them I'm with you. Tell them I'm right here in the bed. Right here. Tell them I'm at home."

"Okay," she said. She swallowed one last time and answered. "Hello," she said.

"Make sure they know," said Ralph. He made sure the tea was clear of his feet and then he let himself fall backward onto the bed, arms spread wide, legs kicking. He hit the bed with a splash. "I'm right here," he mumbled. "I'm at home."

INTERVIEW: MARIA BAMFORD

DO YOU HAVE ANY ROUTINES OR REMEDIES FOR WHEN YOU CAN'T SLEEP?

Maria Bamford: Reading, stretching, graham crackers and milk, tubs and then, if all else fails, Tylenol PM or Seroquel.

WHAT HAVE YOU LOST THE MOST SLEEP OVER IN YOUR LIFE?

Maria Bamford: I am Bipolar II and so I have episodes of High Anxiety followed by long periods of Depression—so, many times I haven't been able to sleep for all of the ruminations on a variety of subjects. Anything will do—relationships of all types (from Singh the Liquor Store Clerk to Match.com winks), money, creative ideas, regret, buying a ceiling fan, cognitive behavioral puzzles, emotional Sudoku. Just last night, post two shows on the road, I couldn't sleep at all after meditating, peanuts, milk, and stretching and so, at 4 AM, I just took a Seroquel (mood stabilizer with sedative effects). I can obsess about anything. Including this question.

DO YOU HAVE ANY RECURRING DREAMS OR THEMES THAT POP UP REGULARLY?

Maria Bamford: Hmm. Nightmares regarding things I haven't done that have caused terrible consequences. Hard to remember, but I wake up a bit sweaty.

WHERE'S THE STRANGEST PLACE YOU'VE EVER SLEPT?

Maria Bamford: I used to be able to sleep anywhere—up against a wall in an airport, in a van filled with comedians farting—but now I am more of a delicate lotus.

IT DARKENS, BROTHER

JIM JOYCE

It begins with my older brother, Colin, who enjoys science fiction, the symphonies of Gustav Mahler, and who has always carried about him a casual sadism.

One night in the early 90s when we were kids, Colin waited until the lights went out and

said, "You know what?"

And I said, "What?"

"Have you ever tried finding that exact moment when you stop being awake and start being asleep?"

"Nope."

"Well you should because when you die it's going to be the same thing."

I sat up in my bed. "No it won't."

"Yes it will," he said. And soon he was asleep, and I was not.

★ ★ ★

At one time, I thought I could find that moment between consciousness and sleep, and conquer it. Only you can't tell exactly at which point you're falling asleep just like you can't tell at which degree water burns skin. It's just different types of heat until you tear your hand away, swearing. Since then, pardoning physical exhaustion or drunkenness, I've had problems getting to sleep, because I keep thinking I'm going to die.

But it doesn't make much sense for a kid to think about dying. In every other part of my life, I was bang my head on cement stupid; I didn't even wear a bike helmet. Still, on the

way to Catholic school, I strolled past the casket factory. So I'm always seeing this deathbox warehouse with its sparks and smoke roar. And I'm spending my formative years at a school that rules with a crucifix heart. It's the type of learning institution that's got a vampire lust for phrases like Most Precious Blood gouged into concrete and an agonized Jesus bleeding eternally in every room.

★ ★ ★

I'm up at 4 a.m., I get five hours of sleep, and now it's time for breakfast. I crack two eggs, slip one yolk into the trash, pour the coffee. It's still dark out. I don't care for that a bit. I pepper the eggs and slouch near the space heater and review my notes for the day.

If I look outside my window, I'll see that my elderly neighbor and fellow early riser, Ms. Ruiz, has already thrown cheerios, spaghetti noodles, and bread onto the square of sidewalk beneath her window for the pigeons and rats to breakfast on.

★ ★ ★

Sleep is the brother of death, at least according to the Greeks, who seemed to know all things first.

Hypnos and Thanatos were their names. They were twin brothers. Do you think they got along well? In the painting by John William Waterhouse, "Sleep and his Half-brother Death," they're drowsing on a Mediterranean couch, Death in the shade, Sleep in the light, and Sleep's just got some poppies loose in his hand. Anyone could pass by and steal those poppies. The two have the unconscious glow and platonic affection of children, androgynous and with hands slung around each other.

Was one ever mistaken for the other during significant moments? Doesn't it seem unfair that something so pleasant as sleep has to be akin to something so presumably unpleasant as death?

★ ★ ★

That I keep thinking I'm going to die any evening now seems stupid, or at least unlikely—young white men don't often die in their sleep. Young white men probably have the lowest mortality rate on the planet, probably at the expense of everyone else's increased mortality.

And anyhow, of course I'm going to die. Thing is, it's inconvenient to think about death all day with the rising dreads at night.

So when I was about seven, I would sigh and moan lowly to myself until I couldn't think and left my bed to meet my mom in the kitchen. She chain-smoked by oven light. Between the two of us and ecclesial smoke twirls, we agreed death was unfair and the best thing was to try not to think about it. And pray and be nice to people. Goodnight.

Because it seems like bad manners, I stopped sighing in bed, but I started tooth grinding, and

all because of the clock tick of death that my brother set off in me.

★ ★ ★

My friend Natalia is deeply spiritual. And religious, too, which is to say she follows the rules and enters church buildings on a regular basis. Natalia also has more nightmares than anyone I've ever met. They are largely apocalyptic and involve invading alien forces and vast destruction, and this from the mind of a woman who does not watch TV or the movies.

Natalia tells me that at the climax of her nightmares there is the feeling that she has been ripped off and the investment in God seems poorly planned. But in the morning, she weighs terror against love and chooses to stay with belief.

One recalls Psalms: "You will not fear the terror of the night, nor the arrow that flies by day." One recalls Proverbs: "If you lie down, you will not be afraid; when you lie down, your sleep will be sweet." Who among us inhabits the relaxed "you" of these aphorisms?

Valiant Natalia – Driver of cars/strummer of guitars! Coax me toward accepting my death!

★ ★ ★

When I was old enough to know better, we were in Theology class at St. Rita HS, and I learned that long ago God switched from a system of works to a system of faith. And I thought, *I am fucked*, and folded my hands over my eyes.

I went to confession that month and explained my situation to a priest through a screen. "I'm a nice guy, mostly, but I don't know if I believe in God."

"How can you see a sunrise and not believe in God?" asked the priest.

And I thought, *You are not helping me.*

And then ten years later there's Natalia, and she's telling me that I have a unique moment, that I have more in common with six billion people than anyone else who has died before me. "Think of all that we have in common!" she says.

★ ★ ★

Sleep has been afflicted for centuries, and not only in the realm of the material world. Civilization has long suffered under the incubus, a monster who rests on the bodies of sleepers.

"Incubus" appears around 1200, meaning "nightmare, one who lies down on [the sleeper]." "Nightmare" appears in the late 13th century as "an evil female spirit afflicting sleepers with a feeling of suffocation," with "Sense of 'any bad dream' first recorded 1829; that of 'very distressing experience' is from 1831."

The word "Incubate" appears later in the 1640s, meaning "To brood upon, watch jealously." In 1721 it appears as "to sit on eggs to hatch them," or "to lie in or upon."

My double bed is an incubator for dark thinking.

★ ★ ★

There was a year when my death watching became unbearable; I'm going to say 2007, when I was 22. Gray thunder of oceans reminded me of death. Washington Square with jugglers and Manhattan trees and jumbo pretzels reminded me of death. The activists I lived with, monastic, dumpstering bagels & watching genocide documentaries full-screened on the computer—they especially made me think about dying.

At 22 I worked around the philosophy section of the university library, second floor north east corner, where people go to get nothing done. It's the meeting place of the Librarian Chess Club, where weary shelvers congregate to drink Crown Royal on the sly, and play a little chess.

While I read a line, "And when you look for a long time into an abyss, the abyss also looks into you," Charlie my coworker was a table over, stretching his arms to me. "Jimmy, put down the books," he unstacked some Dixie cups, filled one halfway. "Play some of this chess with us."

★ ★ ★

At 22, each day became a black t-shirt day. When my friend Monica left her black nail polish on the coffee table in our apartment, it went to use.

At the coffeeshop, I drew skulls and ghosts all over receipt paper and coffee cups. My boss asked what the hell was my problem. I told him I was in a gang and this was the only way to get new members.

He didn't bat an eye. "Good," he said, "maybe they can teach you to be more disciplined. You forgot to take out the garbage last night."

Next day at work, in the back office I saw a bottle of nail polish remover resting on top of a five-dollar bill. The bill and bottle each bore a message in black Sharpie. "HAIRCUT," said the bill. "NO MORE CRYIN," said the bottle.

★ ★ ★

Public Service Announcement from the head of the mathematics department: "Statistically speaking, humans are more likely to be alive than dead. You are more likely to live than to die." For how long? We don't know. But at this moment there are more people inhabiting the planet—eating cookies in bed, getting off at the wrong bus stop, picking fruit, misreading text messages—than at any other time in history. Taking the mathematical view, death is unlikely.

Other times there is no announcement in my office, and I walk in to see the math teacher is lying on the floor. Uh oh, I think.

"I'm just stretching my bad back," he says. "Walk around me, go on. And promise me something."

"Anything," I say, hoping it's easy.

"Don't ever get old," he says, rising. "It sucks."

★ ★ ★

If you've got a few bucks, the 21st century allows for easier sleeping. There are exterminators for vermin, there is internal heat and air conditioning, and a highly flammable comforter can be purchased for around $20 at most department stores. And for those who are difficult to love, there is even the hug-a-pillow, which recreates the human form in the shape of a crescent moon for harmless spooning.

My boss at the UIC writing center, Vaynus, told me that in Lithuanian summers prior to the industrial revolution, families slept under sheets soaked in cold water. More homes outside of major urban areas were built half submerged in earth or dug into hillsides. And it wasn't until the 20th century that fleas and bedbugs were evicted from the bedroom; up until then, even kings and queens had fleas.

★ ★ ★

In paintings, the incubus is seen either lying prostrate over a sleeper, or sitting hunched on the sleeper's chest—see Fuseli's "Nightmare." What's this ghost monster's agenda? Reportedly, he robs the semen of men (detailed reports desired) and uses it to conceive with a woman. St. Augustine, in his book *City of God*, had to throw up his hands in weariness at the number of incubi assaults. There were so many reports "…which trustworthy persons who have heard the experience of others corroborate… that it were impudent to deny [their existence.]" Augustine's predecessor, St. Thomas of Aquinas, would return to this topic and explain, with the cold logic of a man convinced, that children born from these couplings were mortal, but with increased powers, like exceptional beauty and immodest ambition.

Who were these power babies? To name a few: "Romulus and Remus, Plato, and Alexander the Great." Are you handsome? Are you ambitious? You might be the product of supernatural union.

★ ★ ★

Faith is dying all around us. My friend Brett works construction, and when the boss is away, half of the team drifts off task. Someone cracks open a Carlsberg beer and passes the bottle around. Things appear: hunks of bread, a bottle of ketchup, salami rolls.

Then the boss's car pulls in view of the window out front. Half-filled bottles are flung out of second story windows, caulk guns spit madly, a powersaw sings to life and snaps scrapwood in half, splinters fly; grown men hammer nails where no nails must go.

When I wake up in the morning it's as though I'm catching my body off guard and its laborers have tumbled into hopeless action. They want to

stay employed. But all I can think about is being hit by a car on the way to work, or the need to buy a security alarm for the rear window. I grow deeply conservative in the early morning.

★ ★ ★

Not to be outdone by St. Augustine or St. Aquinas, Pope Sylvester II (999-1003) admitted to repeated relations with a female incubus, though the encounters were prior to his papacy. He revealed this on his deathbed, needing to get the affair off his chest and die repentant. But this might not be reliable. Reports of his death vary wildly. One involves a devil stealing Pope Sylvester's eyes, another reports that the devil never left his side, padding along in the form of a black dog.

A heavy conscience, deocculization, stalwart dogs: all of these things make rest difficult.

★ ★ ★

Marco is a talented tattoo artist in Oak Park. Nine years ago I sat in his old Ashland studio while my friend Erik got tattooed. Over the buzz of the needle and between gentle wipes with the blood rag, Marco told us how his house was haunted. With sexy ghosts.

"I'm not kiddin you guys. It's happened twice," he said. "This ghost is screwing me in my sleep. I wake up, you know, at the big moment," he made a slow explosion gesture

with his hand, "and this warm figure is floating over me. And just what the hell am I supposed to do?"

We shrugged.

"And I got my kid in the other room. I mean, do I tell him about it?"

We shook our heads.

★ ★ ★

In defense of immortality, there is the appeal of nostalgia and the passing of things I might miss. Like my body, which I use every day. Or cherry cola, which pours endlessly from movie theater fountains. But can you be nostalgic for people, or does the mind accept death? Can I have nostalgia for dead loved ones?

I am not nostalgic for my Grandma. I miss her, but I respect her death, too. Maybe a grave is a picture frame. After the pain, her death helped me see her as a person completed and for once understandable.

★ ★ ★

I'm scared of many things, like not doing my job well. Taxes frighten me, and so does removing my wisdom teeth. I don't want to get hit by a car again either, though I'm steeling myself for it.

Louis Ferdinand Celine, ellipses master and author doctor, he got kicked out of France for being an alleged Nazi collaborator. He wrote on dread and anxiety, too. "Never believe straight

off in a man's unhappiness," notes Celine. "Ask him if he can still sleep. If the answer's 'yes,' all's well. That is enough."

I almost fall asleep fine as an adult, but when I wake after about five hours of sleep, I think about dying. With each day's blooming moment, I'm shaking my head and imagining the bus that will finally crush my bike asunder, or the mugging in a strange city that'll leave me on a bench, blood drained.

★ ★ ★

I've predicted a forecast for my travelling anxiety. My theory, which is uninformed, says that in five more years there will be some sort of dread leaving my evenings and passing into the afternoon, unfolding over me like overcast weather while I'm at work. Maybe it's already started.

Last week we were reading a Marquez short story about a dentist who works without Novocain. A kid started asking about unreliable narrators when a stray sparrow slammed into the classroom window. It hit it so hard the room thumped like a bass drum.

Chairs squeaked.

"Wow!" said one kid, slamming his palm on the desk.

"Oh, Mylanta! That's so awful," said another.

Everyone looked at me. I had nothing to give them.

★ ★ ★

All dreams are shitty metaphors. You're lost at sea. You're naked in front of the classroom. Got it. But what about this: once I dreamed my friend Doug became a famous painter. He took me to his studio for a dinner party. When I turned in a crowd to greet him I spilled my wine glass on the prettiest woman in the room. I stared, humiliated. Doug tried to change the subject and pointed to a mural on his wall. I found that I liked it. When I woke up, I drew the mural from memory in my notebook. I saw Doug for lunch.

"Take it, it's your artwork," I said.

My dream made me the owner of that painting, but only as a British archeologist is the owner of a grave-robbed Egyptian mummy. I wished Doug would have gotten more excited about my discovery of his work—entered it in contests and turned it into a handbag for young art students to buy from Blick on State street.

Then I could go on TV or blogs and say, "Certainly it is his drawing, but did I not discover it?"

Nothing happened. Doug made some details with a pen and slipped it into his wallet in a way that didn't put our friendship in jeopardy. I'm compelled to embellish this story should I tell it again. Why do I remember this dream?

★ ★ ★

I like the Old Testament with its portentous evenings and sledgehammer justice, relighting dying fires, falling-down-a-well deaths and swinging ass's jaws. I understand violence. It's peace and kindness and patience that confound me.

Sometimes I wonder what would it be like to have a modern day interpreter of dreams, like Joseph Son of Jacob. Between my brother and fourteen years of Catholic school, I have an obsession for the morbid and gothic, but no way of reading the details. There remains the need for explanation.

The lack of dream readers and decoders must be why so many Irish and Mexican kids turn toward The Misfits, Bauhaus, The Smiths, and Morrissey. So many lyrics about dying all the time but never being dead, so many two minutes and fifty-nine second monster songs.

★ ★ ★

All of my black band t-shirts are gray from over-washing. I'm mellowing now, and I write short songs under a minute thirty seconds like verse/chorus/bridge and wear white shirts and red sneakers. My zines get shorter, too.

When I am the master of my form, I'll just write fortunes for the cookies in Chinese restaurants. The best one I've ever read says, "It's time to sleep; I'm going to dream now."

CONTRIBUTORS' NOTES

Tara Abbamondi is a cartoonist/illustrator/comics-making lady. Currently she is working on multiple anthology pieces and two full-length comics. She lives in the woods with her husband, Paul. She can sleep in anything but silence.

J. Adams Oaks is the author of the Booklist-starred novel, *WHY I FIGHT* (A Richard Jackson Book, Simon and Schuster), a Junior Library Guild Selection and award winner from the National Society of Arts and Letters, Friends of American Writers, Illinois Arts Council, and is included in the 2010 ALA Best Books For Young Adults and Texas TAYSHAS Reading List. His short fiction has appeared in *River Oak Review, Cellstories, The Madison Review, The Nervous Breakdown* and *Windy City Queer Anthology,* as well as being featured on Chicago Public Radio. When he isn't sound asleep with too many pillows and his dog at his feet, he's hard at work on his second novel.

James Tadd Adcox's first book, *The Map of the System of Human Knowledge*, a short fictional encyclopedia of everything, is available from Tiny Hardcore Press. He sleeps like death.

Lauryn Allison Lewis writes fiction, essays, interviews, and reviews of all sorts. She is a managing editor at Curbside Splendor Press, and an assistant editor at Barrelhouse Magazine. Lauryn's novella, *solo/down,* was published in 2012 by The Chicago Center for Literature and Photography, and her debut novel, *The Beauties,* will be published later this year by Silverthought Press.

Andrew Bales' stories have appeared in *New Delta Review*, *Midwestern Gothic*, *Johnny America*, and *NANO Fiction*, among others, and have received second-place in *Glimmer Train's* Short Story Award for New Writers. "I am the Sea Captain, I am Lance Armstrong, I am Tonya Harding" was Runner-Up in *Beecher's* First Annual Fiction Contest, judged by Deb Olin Unferth. Andrew lives in Wichita, Kansas, with his girlfriend. When she is out of town, he lies diagonally, because why not, and swears the moon stalks him as he sleeps.

Pamela Balluck's creative writing has appeared in, among other publications, *Western Humanities Review*, *The Southeast Review*, *Quarter After Eight*, *Square Lake*, *Jabberwock Review*, *Barrow Street*, *Night Train*, *Freight Stories*, *Avery Anthology*, *Prime Mincer* and is forthcoming in *Robert Olen Butler Prize Stories* and in *The Ocean State Review*. Balluck teaches writing at the University of Utah. She is still searching for the optimal setting on her Sleep Number® Bed.

Maria Bamford is the first female comedian to have two half-hour *Comedy Central Presents* specials. She starred in the film and Comedy Central series *The Comedians of Comedy* and contributes comedic voiceovers for several animations including PBS's Emmy-winning series *Word Girl*. Her one-woman web series *The Maria Bamford Show* was featured at the Museum of Arts and Design in New York, and her 2009 CD *Unwanted Thoughts Syndrome* was named one of the best comedy albums of the decade by The Onion's The AV Club. Maria jerks wildly in her sleep at irregular intervals due to caffeine use.

Ron Barrett was born in the Bronx, New York. His comic strips, *Politenessman*, *Dog Date Diary*, *I Date the Great*, *The Masked Doctor and the Secret Nurse* and *Steve Draper, Custom Reupholsterer* appeared in *The National Lampoon* when it was really good. Ron later became the magazine's art director and funeral director. He removes his shoes before going to bed and wears a necktie with his pajamas.

Angi Becker Stevens' stories have appeared in a variety of publications including *The Collagist*, *Pank*, *Monkeybicycle*, *Wigleaf*, *SmokeLong Quarterly*, *Knee-Jerk*, *Barrelhouse*, *30 Under 30*, and *Best of the Web 2010*. Her debut fiction collection, *All I Ever Learned From Love*, is forthcoming from Aqueous Books in early 2014. She sleeps reluctantly, long after midnight.

Nick Bertozzi is the Harvey Award-winning author of *Lewis and Clark* (First Second) and *The Salon* (St Martin's Press), a graphic novel about Picasso and magical absinthe. He has collaborated with Jason Lutes on the cartoon-biography *Houdini: The Handcuff King* (Hyperion). He has been teaching cartooning at NYC's School of Visual Arts, lives in NYC with his wife and daughters, and he sleeps with his feet hanging over the bed.

Jeffrey Brown is a Chicago cartoonist known for his autobiographical graphic novel (*Clumsy, Funny Misshapen Body*) and humorous comics (*Incredible Change-Bots, Cats Are Weird*). He sometimes finds himself sleeping with his four year old son's feet kicking him in the head.

Joey Comeau is a firm believer in the idea that if you can't be a good example, you have an obligation to be a horrible warning. He writes the comic *A Softer World*. He has a degree in linguistics which really only comes in handy when smart-asses try to correct his grammar at parties. He really, really likes candy. Like, sour candies mostly. Fuzzy peaches. Sour grapes. But man, yeah. Candy. Joey doesn't sleep so good.

Hugh Crawford is a creator of the daily comic strip, *Crimes Against Hugh's Manatees*. He lives in Joplin, Missouri with his wife and two daughters. Hugh sleeps soundly, except on the nights when the fear of dying in his sleep keeps him up.

Winner of the One Book, One Chicago flash fiction writing contest, **Robert Duffer**'s (robertduffer. com) work has appeared in *Chicago Tribune, MAKE Magazine, Chicago Reader, Knee-Jerk Magazine, Time Out Chicago, Monkeybicycle, Chicago Public Radio, Annalemma, New City, Flashquake*, and other coffee-table favorites like *Canadian Builders Quarterly*. He edits a Sunday column on fatherhood (experimentsinmanhood.com), and recently set a personal record as a parent by sleeping for seven uninterrupted hours. On good nights, he sleeps with his wife.

Natalie Edwards' fiction has appeared in the *Chicago Reader, McSweeney's Internet Tendency, decomP, Untoward, Another Chicago Magazine*, on *the Rumpus*, and, you know, around here and there. The Rumpus named her one of the funniest women of *McSweeney's*, and she is the editor of the featherproof minibook series. You can read and hear more at natalieaedwards.com. She sleeps 20 minutes longer than she should, but always manages to get there on time.

Roxane Gay lives and writes in the Midwest. She does not get nearly enough sleep.

Rick Geary has been a freelance cartoonist and illustrator for 38 years. His illustrations and graphic stories have appeared in *National Lampoon, MAD, The New York Times, Heavy Metal, Disney Adventures* and many other publications. His graphic novels include the biographies *J. Edgar Hoover* and *Trotsky,* as well as nine volumes in the series "A Treasury of Victorian Murder," and four volumes in "A Treasury of 20th Century Murder," the latest of which is *The Lives of Sacco & Vanzetti*. Rick and his wife Deborah live in Carrizozo,

New Mexico. See more of his work at rickgeary.com. Rick says, "My favorite thing about sleeping is that I'm generally able to drop off right away. My least favorite thing is that I rarely remember my dreams."

Sharon Goldner's stories (over 30) have been published in literary journals all over the place, including forthcoming in a HarperCollins anthology. She is a 3-time Pushcart Prize nominee. Additionally, her plays have been produced in NYC, Baltimore, and in Florida. Sharon's favorite sleep thing is when she dreams of flying, and though it takes her a few tries, she eventually makes it up in the air and is soaring, birds and Superman be damned.

Eric Haven is the creator of the comics *Tales to Demolish*, *The Aviatrix*, and *Race Murdock*. He's also the blueprint cartoonist for the TV show *MythBusters*. At any given moment, Eric's not entirely sure if he's awake or lucid dreaming.

Cynthia Hawkins is a freelance writer, educator, and Associate Editor of Arts and Culture for *The Nervous Breakdown*. Her work has appeared in publications such as *ESPN the Magazine*, *Monkeybicycle*, and *Passages North*. She once fell asleep during a showing of *Ordinary Decent Criminal* in a London cinema (someone please tell her how it ends).

David Heatley is a cartoonist and musician who lives in Queens with his wife (the writer, Rebecca Gopoian) and their two children. His critically acclaimed graphic memoir *My Brain is Hanging Upside Down* has been translated into 3 other languages and was called by the *NY Times Book Review* "a beautifully unsettling mosaic of comic-strip jokes." Heatley has been writing, performing and recording music since 1992. His band, The Bischoffs, plays frequently in the NYC area. He is often asleep five minutes after his head hits the pillow.

Owen Heitmann is an award-winning cartoonist based in South Australia. His credits include comics and zines such as *How To Save The World: A Beginner's Guide* (a 48-page zombie comic self-published with the aid of a grant from the South Australian Youth Arts Board), *Last Night* (a 24-hour comic), and *Stamp Out Evil* (with Evil Dan), as well as the webcomics *Outta My Head*, *Basic Wage Kids* and *5031* (all available online at 24hourcynic.com). He has contributed to numerous Australian and international comics anthologies, and has written about comics for *The Weekend Australian*, the *Sydney Morning Herald*, *The Age*, *Rip It Up* magazine, *Excitement Machine* and *OzComics Magazine*. He prefers to sleep wearing earplugs.

Steve Himmer is the author of the novel The Bee-Loud Glade, and the ebook short The Second Most Dangerous Job In America. He edits the webjournal *Necessary Fiction*, and lives outside Boston. He has never been a very good sleeper.

Nathan Holic is the Graphic Narrative Editor at *The Florida Review*, and the series editor of *15 Views of Orlando* (Burrow Press). Though he sometimes draws traditional comics and writes traditional prose, his work most often drifts between different forms, with short stories incorporating comics or Wikipedia pages or flipbooks. You can read his ongoing comic series "Clutter" (a comic structured as a home decor catalogue) at *Smalldoggies Magazine* online, and you can find Nathan at nathanholic.com. He has not slept since January 5, 2012, the day on which his son Jackson was born.

Emily Horne has lived in all the oceanfront provincial capitals except St John's Newfoundland. She grew up near Charlottetown, Prince Edward Island, went to University in Halifax, Nova Scotia and fled for five years to Victoria, British Columbia. Now she's joined Joey in Toronto, where she takes the photos for *A Softer World*, designs the comic, and wonders when things will get better. Emily sleeps with her hands above her head, even though she thought she heard somewhere that it's bad...

William Hughes is a writer of short humorous fiction and his own (mostly illegible) signature. His work has appeared in *McSweeney's* and on a wide variety of credit card receipts. He sleeps on a waterbed purchased in a more innocent, less aware-of-how-uncomfortable-waterbeds-are time.

Tim Jones-Yelvington is a Chicago-based writer and multimedia performance artist. He is the author of "Evan's House and the Other Boys who Live There" (in *They Could No Longer Contain Themselves*, Rose Metal Press) and *This is a Dance Movie!* (Tiny Hardcore Press, forthcoming). His work has appeared in *Harpur Palate, Puerto del Sol, Another Chicago Magazine* and others. He guest edits *[PANK]*'s annual Queer issue. He smacks his lips in his sleep.

Jim Joyce is a high school English teacher in Chicago. His writing has appeared in *Mildred Pierce, Chicago Tribune*, and his zine, *Or Let It Sink*. Jim goes to bed at 10 and gets up at 4. He drools in his sleep.

Kenny Keil is an artist and writer living in Los Angeles with his wife and son. He still sleeps with a blanket his mom made for him when he was in junior high.

Michael Koh lives in Buffalo, New York. He gets kicked sometimes by Annie when sleeping, so he hogs the covers.

Etgar Keret is an Israeli writer and filmmaker. His writing has been published in *The New Yorker*, the *New York Times, Harper's Magazine* and *The Paris Review*. "Jellyfish," his first movie as a director along with his wife, Shira Geffen, won the Camera d'Or prize for best first feature at Cannes in 2007. In 2010 he was named a Chevalier of France's Order of Arts and Letters. His latest collection of short stories, *Suddenly a Knock on the Door*, came out in English last March. From a very young age he'd wake up with some incomplete memories of a dreams and make up stories out of them. By the time he was old enough to know he's supposed to analyze the dreams and not write stories out of them it was already too late.

Todd Levin was a writer for *Late Night with Conan O'Brien, The Tonight Show with Conan O'Brien* (remember that???), and *The Onion News Network*. His writing has also been published in a number of magazines and books. He co-authored the humor book, *SEX: Our Bodies, Our Junk*, available now from Broadway/Random House. He sleeps soundly, with the help of an adorable dental night guard, although the sleeping position he find most comfortable is also pretty spooky to witness: lying on his back, with his hands crossed over his heart, like Bela Lugosi in *Dracula*.

Susan L. Lin studied creative writing and studio art at the University of Houston. Her work has recently appeared in *Poet Lore, elimae*, and *Rougarou*. She has been an insomniac since childhood.

Billy Lombardo is the Co-Founder/Managing Editor of *Polyphony H.S.*, an int'l, student-run litmag for high school writers/editors. He is the author, most recently, of *The Man with Two Arms* (novel)*,* and the forthcoming YA novel, *Homeschool Steffie: The Day of the Palindrome*. Billy won the Nelson Algren Award for the Short Story in 2011. He teaches at the Latin School of Chicago and is the 2012-23 Writer-in-Residence at Roosevelt University. In the summer he sleeps with his left hand in his boxers. In the winter he wears sleeping pants.

Joe Lo Truglio is an actor/writer who began his career as a founding member of the cult sketch group *The State*. He has appeared in the movies *Superbad, Role Models, Paul*, and *Wet Hot American Summer*, among others. He loves horror movies and, according to his dentist, has been known to grind his teeth when he sleeps.

Rachel Mans is a 2006 Presidential Scholar in the Arts. She graduated from Creighton University in 2009 with a degree in creative writing and from Iowa State University in 2012 with an MA in Literature. A 2005 alumna of the Pennsylvania Governor's School for the Arts, which was financially disbanded and now rests in peace, she has published in *Shadows* and *Knee-Jerk*. She sleeps under a quilt that her mother made for her, on her stomach and as still as a stone.

Becky Margolis has an MFA from the University of Montana. Some of her stories can be found in *Necessary Fiction, Umbrella Factory Magazine*, and the *Prism Review*. She lives in Missoula, where she counts bears to sleep.

T.J. Miller is an improvisation, sketch, and stand-up comedian and actor who has appeared in the films *Get Him to the Greek, Colverfield, Our Idiot Brother,* and *Seeking a Friend at the End of the World* among others. He was named one of *Variety*'s Top 10 Comics to Watch as well as one of *Entertainment Weekly*'s Next Big Thing in Comedy. He sleeps on moving vehicles with ease.

Tony Millionaire was born in Boston and grew up in Gloucester, Massachusetts. He writes and draws the ongoing adventures of *Sock Monkey*, published by Dark Horse Comics. He is the creator of the syndicated comic strip, *MAAKIES*, which has been collected by Fantagraphics, who also publishes his graphic novel series, *Billy Hazelnuts*, and his latest book *500 Portraits by Tony Millionaire*. His house is infested with kids, pets, toys, and a beautiful wife. A night worker, he sleeps till 2 PM every day. Around noon he is generally dreaming of young nymphs rustling between the sheets in squatted houses. By 1:30 the dreams turn to bombs, disaster, murder and snakes, so he jumps out of bed.

Jimmy Pardo is the host of the award-winning podcast *Never Not Funny* and the official opening act for Conan O'Brien at *Conan* tapings. He is the star of his own half-hour *Comedy Central Presents* special and has performed on *The Tonight Show with Jay Leno* and *The Late Late Show with Craig Ferguson*. Jimmy hosted GSN's *National Lampoon's Funny Money* and co-hosted four seasons of AMC's *Movies at Our House*. He also hosted episodes of VH1's *The Surreal Life, Love Lounge* and NBC's *Late Friday*. Jimmy Pardo hasn't had a good night's sleep in over 40 years!

Margaret Patton Chapman teaches writing at Indiana University South Bend and is fiction editor at *decomP magazinE*. Her fiction has been published in *decomP, Kill Author, Diagram, elimae, The 2ndhand*, and as a Featherproof mini-book. Recently, she's been sleeping in fits and starts, but still, when she does sleep, she almost always has enjoyable dreams.

Jesse Reklaw has been drawing the weekly comic strip *Slow Wave* since 1995. He does some other stuff too, and is working on a comics memoir to be published in a year or two, he hopes. His other books are *Dreamtoons* and *The Night of Your life* (both are illustrated dreams), and *Applicant* and *Ten Thousand Things to Do*. He often sleeps while spooning his cat, Littles.

Credited with pioneering efforts in the worlds of music, video, performance art and multimedia, **The Residents** have fascinated audiences with their daring and imagination for four decades. During that time they have released over 50 albums, countless videos and DVDs and toured the world seven times. In 2006 they were honored with a career retrospective of their video work at the Museum of Modern Art in New York. Since the group has zealously protected its privacy beneath a blanket of anonymity, little is known about their sleeping habits, but Randy, the Residents' longtime singer and front man is rumored to be an avid napper, especially when touring.

Mary Roach is the author of the New York Times bestsellers *Packing for Mars: The Curious Science of Life in the Void*; *Stiff: The Curious Lives of Human Cadavers*; *Bonk: The Curious Coupling of Science and Sex*; and *Spook: Science Tackles the Afterlife*. *Packing for Mars* is a New York Times Editor's Choice and was chosen as the San Francisco 2011 One City, One Book selection. *Stiff* has been translated into 17 languages, and *Spook* was a New York Times Notable Book. Mary has written for *National Geographic, Wired, New Scientist, The New York Times Book Review, the Journal of Clinical Anatomy*, and *Outside*, among others. She is a member of the Mars Institute's Advisory Board and the guest editor of the 2011 *Best American Science and Nature Writing*. She sleeps in hunting socks.

Bryan Rubio is a dreamer. As a child living in a trailer park commune, he dreamt of freedom. As a teen wishing for the attention of the fairer sex, he dreamt of popularity. As a struggling musician in his early twenties, he dreamt of rock stardom. Now, as a man closing in on 40, his dream is to be able to sleep an entire night without being kicked out of his own bed by his two children.

Matthew Salesses is the author of *The Last Repatriate* (Nouvella, 2011) and two chapbooks, *Our Island of Epidemics* [PANK] and *We Will Take What We Can Get* (Publishing Genius). His stories have or will appear in *Glimmer Train, Witness, American Short Fiction, The Literary Review, West Branch,* and others. He writes a column and edits fiction for the *Good Men Project*. He sleeps when his baby sleeps, which is never often enough.

Dakota Sexton writes about art, oddball culture, travel, and sustainability, and will—on occasion—elaborate on her obsession with typography and her past life as a child historical re-enactor. She holds

a BFA in creative writing from Columbia College, and works as the web editor of *Yoga International* magazine. She will bogart your covers. (That's a promise.)

Michael Showalter was a founding member of the sketch comedy troupe, *The State*, which ran for three seasons on MTV. Michael is also a member of the comedy trio Stella, and, along with Michael Ian Black and David Wain, starred in its eponymous Comedy Central series. He co-wrote, co-produced and starred in the cult comedy *Wet Hot American Summer* and directed, wrote and starred in the *The Baxter* co-starring Michelle Williams, Elizabeth Banks and Justin Theroux. His stand-up comedy record, *Sandwiches & Cats* was released in 2007 (JDub Records). Michael and longtime collaborator Michael Ian Black co-wrote, co-directed, and co-starred in a well-acclaimed series for Comedy Central, *Michael and Michael Have Issues*. He also created a popular web interview series on Collegehumor.com called The Michael Showalter Showalter. He teaches screenwriting at NYU Graduate Film School and his comedic memoir, *Mr. Funny Pants*, hit shelves February 24, 2011 (Hachette Book Group). He sleeps with his cats.

Curtis Smith's stories and essays have appeared in over eighty literary journals. His most recent books are *Bad Monkey* (stories, Press 53), *Truth or Something Like It* (novel, Casperian Books), and *Witness* (essays, Sunnyoutside). He is a big fan of sleep. In fact, the first thing he thinks about each morning are his odds of fitting in a nap later in the day.

Simon A. Smith writes and teaches English in Chicago where he lives with his wife and a murderous orange tabby named Cheever. His fiction has appeared or is forthcoming in *Hobart, Quick Fiction, Keyhole, Monkeybicycle, Whiskey Island, [PANK]* and more. He sleeps only after at least two glasses of wine, the covers scissored between his severely outstretched legs, and dreams of high school acquaintants he barely knew at the time...

Megan Stielstra is the author of *Everyone Remain Calm*, a story collection, and the Literary Director of Chicago's 2nd Story storytelling series. She's told stories for The Goodman, The Steppenwolf, The Museum of Contemporary Art, The Neo-Futurarium, Story Week Festival of Writers, and Chicago Public Radio, among others, and performs regularly with 2nd Story, The Paper Machete, and Write Club. Her fiction and essays have appeared in *Other Voices, The Nervous Breakdown, Fresh Yarn, Monkeybicycle, Pindeldyboz, Swink, Necessary Fiction, Annalemma,* and *Punk Planet*, among others, and she currently teaches creative writing at Columbia College and The University of Chicago. Megan lives across the street from the Aragon, a legendary rock club on Chicago's North Side, and has slept through

Rob Zombie, Megadeath, and Marilyn Manson, whose fans broke a tree in front of her building. Marilyn Manson owes her a tree.

Ben Tanzer is the author of the books *You Can Make Him Like You, My Father's House, So Different Now* and *This American Life* among others. He also oversees day-to-day operations of *This Zine Will Change Your Life* and can be found online at *This Blog Will Change Your Life,* the center of his vast, albeit faux media empire. Ben never sleeps, 'cause sleep is the cousin of death.

Sally Jane Thompson (sallyjanethompson.co.uk) is a freelance illustrator and comic creator based in the UK, where she works on both commissioned work and her own stories. She sleeps under the warmest duvet she could find, and only remembers dreams if she wakes up before they're finished.

J. A. Tyler is the author of eight books, including *Variations of a Brother War* and *In Love with a Ghost*. His work has appeared with *Cream City Review, Redivider, Brooklyn Rail, Diagram*, and others. He sleeps beneath a down comforter. To bed with him, clamor through this open window: chokeonthesewords.com.

David Wain is a director, writer and performer, known for such projects as *Wet Hot American Summer, Role Models, The State, Stella* and *Childrens Hospital*. His most recent movie is *Wanderlust* (2012). When his wife woke him because he was snoring loudly one night, he yelled defensively, "That's impossible, I'm not even asleep!" Then he realized his wife would have no motivation to accuse him of snoring if it wasn't true, and he understood what a dumb dumb he is.

Brandi Wells is Managing Editor of *The Black Warrior Review* and Web Editor at *Hobart*. She is the author of *Please Don't Be Upset* (Tiny Hardcore Press) and *Poisonhorse* (Nephew, An imprint of Mudluscious Press). Her fiction can be found in *Salamander, Mid-American Review, 14 Hills* and many other journals. She drools profusely in her sleep and isn't embarrassed about it.

Julia Wertz was born in the bay area in 1982 and now lives in Brooklyn, NY. She's the cartoonist/writer of the unfortunately titled *Fart Party vol 1 & 2* (Atomic Books) and *Drinking at the Movies* (Random House). Her work can be found at juliawertz.com. She still sometimes dreams about the apocalypse, but now it's a lot sexier.

Shannon Wheeler began cartooning for the University of California, Berkeley student newspaper. Later he created *Too Much Coffee Man* which has run as a weekly newspaper comic, a web comic, in

comic books, in magazines and collected in graphic novels. *Too Much Coffee Man* even lays claim to being the first opera based on a comic book. *The New Yorker* began publishing single panel cartoons from Wheeler in 2009. BOOM! published a collection of *New Yorker* submissions in the book *I Thought You Would Be Funnier* (2010). Wheeler is currently working on a graphic novel about the Gulf Coast oil spill. He sleeps a lot less than he would like.

Alison Wight has drawn comics for years and finally started putting them up on sentfromthemoon.com recently. She's also an illustrator and graphic designer, and generally throws herself around Greenpoint, Brooklyn, drawing comics, going to bars, drawing comics in bars, and occasionally dreaming she's doing one thing while she's doing another.

Catriona Wright is a writer and ESL teacher living in Toronto, Canada. She has an MA in Creative Writing from the University of Toronto, and her work has appeared in various Canadian and American literary journals. As a child she used to sleepwalk, but nowadays she just sleeptalks, sleep laughs, and sleepsings.

ALSO BY CURBSIDE SPLENDOR

Chicago Stories: 40 Dramatic Fictions by Michael Czyzniejewski

Piano Rats 44 stories by Franki Elliot

The Chapbook poems by Chares Bane, Jr.

Sophomoric Philosophy a novel by Victor David Giron

MAY WE SHED THESE HUMAN BODIES short stories by Amber Sparks

Curbside Splendor a semi-annual literary journal that celebrates urbanism

Another Chicago Magazine a bi-annual themed literary journal (www.antoherchicagomagazine.net)

New Poems / Nuevos Poemas by Charles Bane Jr. (October 2012; Concepcion Book, a Curbside imprint)

Everything Flows short stories by James Greer (November 2012)

FORTHCOMING

The Waiting Tide poems by Ryan W. Bradley
written as an homage to Pablo Neruda's The Captain's Verses (Spring 2013, Concepcion Books)

The Typewriter Stories by Franki Elliot (Spring 2013)

Life Stories by Chicago writer Samantha Irby (Fall 2013)

Knee-Jerk

a journal of prose, comics, and more

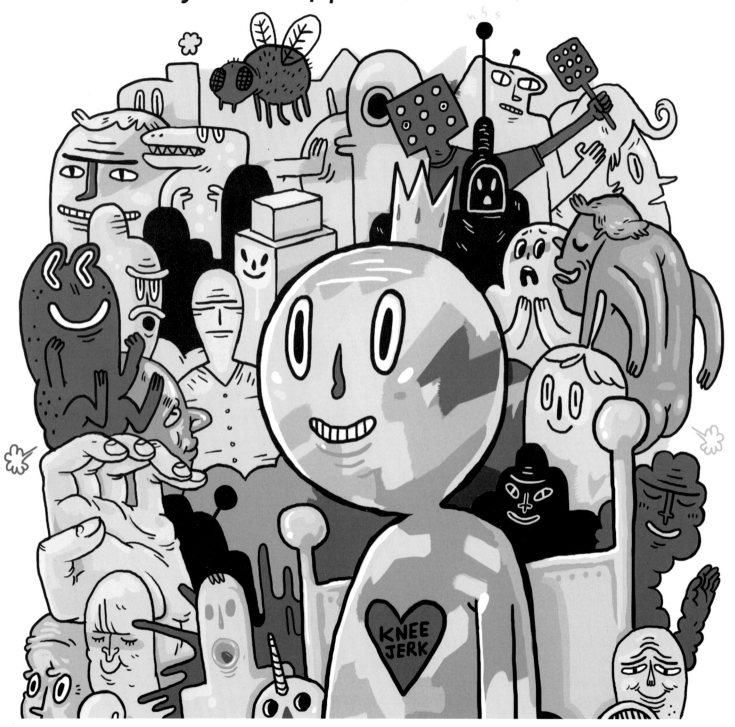

kneejerkmag.com